COVID-19 and Migration: Understanding the Pandemic and Human Mobility

COVID-19
& Migration
Understanding the Pandemic and Human Mobility

Edited by

Ibrahim Sirkeci and Jeffrey H. Cohen

TRANSNATIONAL PRESS LONDON
2020

Migration Series: 23

COVID-19 and Migration: Understanding the Pandemic and
Human Mobility

Edited by Ibrahim Sirkeci and Jeffrey H. Cohen

First Published in 2020 by TRANSNATIONAL PRESS
LONDON in the United Kingdom, 12 Ridgeway Gardens,
London, N6 5XR, UK.
www.tplondon.com

Transnational Press London® and the logo and its affiliated
brands are registered trademarks.

Requests for permission to reproduce material from this work
should be sent to: sales@tplondon.com

Paperback
ISBN: 978-1-912997-59-6
Hardcover
ISBN: 978-1-912997-71-8
Digital
ISBN: 978-1-912997-60-2

Cover Design: Nihal Yazgan
Cover Image: Black vector created by starline - www.freepik.com

www.tplondon.com

CONTENT

i

ABOUT THE AUTHORS

Ibrahim Sirkeci, PhD, is Professor of Transnational Studies and Marketing, Head of Marketing Subject Cluster, Interim Assistant Dean for Research, Leader of PhD Programme and Director of Centre for Transnational Business and Management at Regent's University London, UK. His research focuses on migration, insecurity, labour markets and remittances in the UK, Turkey, Iraq, and Germany. He has authored and edited many books and leads many journals including *Migration Letters* and *Remittances Review*. Ibrahim is also the chair of The Migration Conferences (TMC).

Jeffrey H. Cohen, PhD, is a professor of anthropology at The Ohio State University. His research on migration and economic development in Mexico, the Dominican Republic, Turkey and China includes support from the National Science Foundation, National Geographic Society, the Fulbright program. His books include *The Cultures of Migration: The Global Nature of Contemporary Movement* (2011) written with Ibrahim Sirkeci and named an outstanding title by Choice Reviews for 2012 and *Eating Soup without a Spoon: Anthropological Theory and Method in the Real World* (2015). He is co-editor of the journals *Migration Letters* and *Remittance Reviews* and is completing *The Culture of Migration Handbook* to be published in 2021by Edward Elgar.

Elizabeth J. Anderson is a research specialist at the International Center for Research on Women. She studies gender, health behaviour, and violence epidemiology.

Julia Arnold is Senior Director, Gender and Financial Inclusion at the Center for Financial Inclusion. She leads research on gender transformative approaches to women's financial inclusion.

Mikheil Batiashvili is based at Business and Technology University, Tbilisi, Georgia.

R. B. Bhagat is Professor and Head, Department of Migration and Urban Studies, International Institute for Population Sciences, Mumbai, India. He is also the Chief Editor of Demography India, an official journal of the Indian Association for the Study of Population (IASP).

Rosa Cabecinhas holds a PhD in Social Psychology of Communication and is professor at the Social Sciences Institute, University of Minho, Portugal. She is Head of the PhD Program in Cultural Studies (University of Minho) and her research interests are interdisciplinary, focusing on social memory, prejudice, migration issues and intercultural communication.

Anu E Castaneda is a research manager at the Finnish Institute for Health and Welfare (THL), Equality and Inclusion Unit and an adjunct professor at the University of Helsinki, Department of Psychology and Logopedics. In THL, she

1

leads a research group focusing on the intersection of cultural diversity and health and wellbeing, including health monitoring of migrants and ethnic minorities, improving evidence-based decision-making and service system development. She was involved in the COVID-19 task force formed by the Ministry of Social Affairs and Health and THL during spring 2020. She also works as a clinical psychologist and psychotherapist in her private practice.

Teresita C. Del Rosario has a background in Sociology from Maryknoll College in the Philippines. She pursued her graduate studies in Public Administration from New York University, a second masters degree in Public Administration from the Harvard Kennedy School of Government, and a Master of Arts degree in Social Anthropology from the Harvard University Faculty of Arts and Sciences.

Yuxia Fu, Nanfang College of Sun Yat-Sen University, Guangzhou China.

Sarah Gammage is the Director of Policy and Government relations for Latin America at the Nature Conservancy. She is a feminist economist and member of the International Association for Feminist Economics.

David Gondauri is Associate Professor at Business and Technology University, Tbilisi, Georgia.

Dipti Govil is Assistant Professor, Department of Population Policies and Programmes, International Institute for Population Sciences, Mumbai, India.

Idil Hussein is a researcher at the Finnish Institute for Health and Welfare (THL), Unit for Infectious Disease Control and Vaccinations. She acts as an administrator of the National Infectious Disease Register. She has previously researched tuberculosis knowledge, attitudes and practices among persons of migrant origin in Finland. She is involved in the task force formed by the Ministry of Social Affairs and Health and THL that coordinates multilingual and multichannel communication on COVID-19. Furthermore, she is currently working on her PhD project.

Agnes Igoye is the Deputy National Coordinator Prevention of Trafficking in Persons, Ministry of Internal Affairs, Uganda. She leads efforts to prevent human trafficking through Uganda's national taskforce.

Zikang Lai, Nanfang College of Sun Yat-Sen University, Guangzhou China.

Ling San Lau, MBBS, MPH, is a pediatric doctor and Senior Program Officer for the Program on Forced Migration and Health and the Care and Protection of Children (CPC) Learning Network at Columbia University's Mailman School of Public Health. Her career has spanned clinical medicine, public health and research, with a focus on forced displacement, child health and child protection.

Linda Alfarero Lumayag is Program Coordinator and Senior Lecturer of Politics and Government Studies, Faculty of Social Sciences and Humanities,

Universiti Malaysia Sarawak, Malaysia.

Sadhana Manik is an associate professor in the Department of Geography Education at the University of KwaZulu-Natal in South Africa.

Philip L. Martin is Emeritus Professor in Agricultural Economics at the University of California, Davis, US. Philip is also the co-chair of the Migration Conferences (TMC) and Co-editor of *Remittances Review*.

Liliana Meza González is a senior economist at the Mexican National Institute of Statistics and Geography (INEGI) and a part-time professor at Universidad Iberoamericana in Mexico City, where she teaches at the Masters program on Migration Studies. She is a member of the Mexican National Research System.

Daniel Naujoks is the Interim Director of International Organization and UN Studies Specialization, Lecturer of International and Public Affairs at Columbia University. He is the author of *Migration, Citizenship, and Development. Diasporic Membership Policies and Overseas Indians in the United States* (2013, Oxford University Press).

Selene Gaspar Olvera is a researcher in the Academic Unit of Development Studies, Autonomous University of Zacatecas. She is also a member of the Information System Project on Migration and Development (SIMDE-UAZ), Mexico.

Carla Pederzini Villareal is a Demographer and a full-time professor and researcher at Universidad Iberoamericana, where she teaches at the Masters program on Migration Studies. She served as President of the Mexican Demographic Society (SOMEDE) from 2013 to 2015 and is currently a member of the editorial committee Coyuntura Demográfica.

Patricia Posch is a PhD candidate at the Social Sciences Institute at University of Minho, Portugal and holds a MsC in Culture and Communication (University of Lisbon). She is engaged in researches that focus on matters of cultural and social memory, identity, and representation related to different social groups, aiming to understand their interplay when it comes to multicultural societies.

Reshmi R.S. is Assistant Professor, Department of Migration and Urban Studies, International Institute for Population Sciences, Mumbai, India.

Smriti Rao is Professor, Economics and Global Studies at Assumption University, and Resident Scholar, Women's Studies Research Center, Brandeis University. She studies the intersection of gender and class, particularly in the global South.

Archana K. Roy is Professor, Department of Migration and Urban Studies, International Institute for Population Sciences, Mumbai, India.

Harihar Sahoo is Assistant Professor, Department of Development Studies,

International Institute for Population Sciences, Mumbai, India.

Melissa Siegel is Professor of Migration Studies at Maastricht University and UNU-MERIT in Maastricht, The Netherlands. Melissa is also the co-director of the Maastricht Center for Citizenship, Migration and Development as well as the Chair of the UNU Migration Network.

Natalia Skogberg, PhD, is a research manager at the Finnish Institute for Health and Welfare (THL), Equality and Inclusion Unit. She is involved in research and development projects in the field of migration and holds expertise in health monitoring, evidence-based service development and in chronic diseases and their risk factors among persons of migrant origin. Since autumn 2020, she had taken the lead of the COVID-19 task force formed by the Ministry of Social Affairs and Health and THL. She also leads the Impact of coronavirus epidemic on wellbeing among foreign born population (MigCOVID) Survey.

Frances S. Sutton is a PhD candidate in the Department of Anthropology at The Ohio State University. She received her BA in Anthropology from Kenyon College in Gambier, OH and her MA in Anthropology from The Ohio State University.

Chi Kong Tse, Department of Electronic Engineering, City University of Hong Kong, Hong Kong, China.

Biao Xiang is Professor of Social Anthropology and Fellow of St Hugh's College at the University of Oxford, UK. He is the author of *The Intermediary Trap* (Princeton University Press, forthcoming) and *Global "Body Shopping"* (Princeton University Press, 2007; winner of 2008 Anthony Leeds Prize; Chinese by Peking University Press 2012).

Rodolfo García Zamora is Professor-Researcher in the Academic Unit of Development Studies, Autonomous University of Zacatecas, Zacatecas, Mexico.

Monette Zard, MA, is the director of the Program on Forced Migration and Health at Columbia University's Mailman School of Public Health. She is an expert on forced migration and human rights, and her career has spanned the fields of policy, advocacy and philanthropy.

Choujun Zhan is Professor at School of Computer, South China Normal University, Guangzhou, China.

Haijun Zhang, Department of Computer Science, Harbin Institute of Technology, Shenzhen 518055, China.

CHAPTER 1

INTRODUCTION

Ibrahim Sirkeci and Jeffrey H. Cohen

The COVID-19 pandemic has disrupted every domain of life. Migration and human mobility, in general, are not exceptions. Since March 2020, researchers, policy makers and many others have channeled their efforts to understand this new coronavirus, its impact and prospects. Many scholars were thinking and writing on the pandemic from its onset and many blog essays quickly appeared. One of the earliest peer-reviewed research articles authored by Sirkeci and Yucesahin (2020) focusing on mobility and travel data showed that it was possible to predict the spatial spread and concentration of COVID-19 cases. Not only was this finding crucial to developing appropriate policies and strategies to counter the spread of the virus, it reminded us that the pandemic is a social disease and not simply a biological threat. The contributions in this book should be considered in this regard tackling the social and policy aspects as we leave the biological and medical side to the experts.

Human mobility is responsive to conflict and insecurity as we have discussed elsewhere (Sirkeci, 2009; Sirkeci and Cohen, 2016; Cohen and Sirkeci, 2011; Cohen and Sirkeci, 2016). One of the greatest threats of COVID-19 pandemic arises from the fact that it is a source of (human) insecurity across several domains. While the most obvious health risk is the potential for death; the virus carries many other the risk, not the least of which is the risk of infection and becoming ill. Alongside health insecurity, COVID-19 exacerbates social inequalities and emphasises health related insecurities as not every country, region or locale is equipped with adequate access to health provision, providers and medical care. Such health insecurity and social inequalities are a cause for concern at a national level and for state actors. However, we are interested in the role, health insecurity and social inequality can play as motivators for some to move.

The threat of COVID-19 caused many countries to lock-down regional and international borders while halting all travel and visa services. While the lock-downs were supported as a way to create security and limit the reach of the virus with national borders, it also created a level of insecurity that adversely affected border crossings. At the same time, it results in further

5

insecurity as some feel urged to move either to exploit an opportunity framework (e.g. lower number of guards at certain borders because of self-isolation or lockdowns) or because they are desperate to get away from worst-affected places. Hence, we have seen continued flows in irregular border crossings[1] and some significant growth in certain corridors. For example, in June to October 2020, it was reported that the channel crossings between France and the UK rose nearly fivefold.[2]

Another direct result of the pandemic is the economic downturn characterised by rising unemployment, inflation, and declining wages. Growing job insecurity and overall economic insecurity affect international migration in many respects. First of all, it increases migration pressure in some places. It also affects remittance flows despite some reported resilience witnessed in certain corridors such as in the US-Mexico corridor. The World Bank experts expect a decline in remittances as a likely effect of the pandemic (World Bank, 2020). Such a decline is likely to increase the emigration pressure at receiving end of some corridors.

A further adverse effect of the COVID-19 is increasing xenophobia and anti-immigration sentiment (Deavakumar et al., 2020; Noel, 2020; HRW, 2020). As many (right-wing) political leaders voiced and repeated in the media, the COVID-19 has been labeled as the "foreign virus", "Chinese virus". There is a clear link between human mobility and the spread of such viruses (Sirkeci and Yücesahin, 2020); however, it does not mean migration is the cause. Casual travel, holidays, and business trips constitute the vast majority of international travel and 20 minutes with an infected person in a closed encounter is considered to be enough to catch the virus. Neither becoming an immigrant nor settlement in another country is necessary. Nevertheless, these negative discourses almost always find their way into policymaking and politics as well as into ordinary everyday opinions and attitudes. The relationship between the COVID-19 and racism and discrimination is yet to be studied and established decisively, but this is surely a source of insecurity that will likely influence the decisions to stay, remigrate or return.

It is important to note that while earlier we were focused on migrants and border crossing, there are state-level changes coming too. The political impact of COVID-19 is likely to follow the patterns of earlier crises. The tightening immigration regulations, visa and admission regimes after the 9/11 New York and 7/7 London bombings are now part of the "normal". Increased airport security is similarly so. The restrictions imposed to "tackle"

---

[1] See https://missingmigrants.iom.int/region/mediterranean.
[2] See several reports from the UK here: https://www.bbc.co.uk/news/uk-england-kent-54589736; https://www.bbc.co.uk/news/uk-england-kent-54000755

the pandemic are, therefore, likely to stay with us and become part of the "new normal".

In this collection of works, we have attempted to bring together early interventions from a group of scholars from around the world, reflecting multidisciplinary nature of the impact. We present a number of conceptual and methodological studies as well as country case studies in the first part, the last part of the book comprises shorter opinion pieces from renown scholars of migration studies.

We hope this book will serve as a starting point for those who are interested in furthering the study of migration and diseases.

References

Devakumar, D., Shannon, G., Bhopal, S. S., & Abubakar, I. (2020). Racism and discrimination in COVID-19 responses. *The Lancet*, 395(10231), 1194.

HRW (2020). Covid-19 Fueling Anti-Asian Racism and Xenophobia Worldwide. https://www.hrw.org/news/2020/05/12/covid-19-fueling-anti-asian-racism-and-xenophobia-worldwide Accessed: 03/11/2020

Noel, T. K. (2020). Conflating culture with COVID-19: Xenophobic repercussions of a global pandemic. *Social Sciences & Humanities Open*, 2(1), 100044. https://dx.doi.org/10.1016%2Fj.ssaho.2020.100044

Sirkeci, I., & Yüceşahin, M. M. (2020). Coronavirus and Migration: Analysis of Human Mobility and the Spread of COVID-19. *Migration Letters*, 17(2), 379-398.

The World Bank (2020). Sharpest Decline in Remittances. Washington DC: World Bank. https://www.worldbank.org/en/news/press-release/2020/04/22/world-bank-predicts-sharpest-decline-of-remittances-in-recent-history   Accessed: 20/09/2020.

CHAPTER 2

COVID-19 AND INTERNATIONAL LABOUR MIGRATION IN AGRICULTURE

Philip L. Martin

Introduction

Table 2.1 shows that the number of international migrants more than tripled between 1970 and 2019, from 84 million to 272 million, and that the migrant share of the world's population rose from 2.3 per cent to 3.5 per cent. Over 60 per cent of the world's international migrants are in Asia (84 million migrants) and Europe (82 million), but migrants are a much larger share of Europe's 740 million people, 11 per cent, than they are of Asia's 4.6 billion people, 1.8 per cent. Migrant shares of the regional populations were highest in Oceania, with eight million or 21 per cent migrants among 38 million people, and North America (Canada and US), with 59 million migrants among 370 million people, making migrants 16 per cent of residents.

Table 2.1. International Migrants, 1970-2019

Year	Number of migrants	Migrants as a % of the world's population
1970	84,460,125	2.3
1975	90,368,010	2.2
1980	101,983,149	2.3
1985	113,206,691	2.3
1990	153,011,473	2.9
1995	161,316,895	2.8
2000	173,588,441	2.8
2005	191,615,574	2.9
2010	220,781,909	3.2
2015	248,861,296	3.4
2019	271,642,105	3.5

Migrants move to opportunity. Two-thirds or 176 million international migrants are in the high income countries, and another third are in middle-income developing countries such as Costa Rica, Turkey, or South Africa. There were 13 million migrants or five per cent of the total stock of migrants

9

in low-income countries.

The ILO estimated there were 164 million migrant workers among 258 million international migrants in 2017, which means that 70 per cent of international migrants 15 and older were employed or looking for work in the country to which they moved. The ILO estimated 150 million migrant workers in 2013, suggesting an average increase of 3.5 million international migrant workers a year between 2013 and 2017.

Men were 58 per cent of international migrant workers in 2017. The share of men 15 and older who were in the labour force was 75 per cent for both migrants and natives in destination countries, but the share of international migrant women in the labour force, 64 per cent, was higher than for native women, 48 per cent. These data refer to international migrant workers in all countries. One reason for the higher labour force participation of international migrant women is that many are employed in health, child, and elderly care in industrial countries, and as domestic workers in middle-income developing countries.

Table 2.2. Migrant Workers by Income Level of Countries, 2017

	Low income	Lower middle income	Upper middle income	High income	All
Total workers	292.6	1216.7	1355.9	599.5	3464.7
Total workers in %	8.4	35.1	39.1	17.3	100
Labour force participation rate for total population	75.0	57.4	65.0	60.3	62
Migrant population aged 15+	8.1	27.7	43.6	154.6	234.0
Migrant population aged 15+ in %	3.5	11.8	18.6	66.1	100
Migrants as a proportion of population aged 15+	2.1	1.3	2.1	15.5	4.2
Migrant workers	5.6	16.6	30.5	111.2	163.8
Migrant workers in %	3.4	10.1	18.6	67.9	100
Labour force participation rate for migrant population	68.5	59.9	69.9	71.9	70.0
Migrant workers as a proportion of all workers	1.9	1.4	2.2	18.5	4.7

Note: Number are given in millions for the following categories: Total workers, Migrant population aged 15+, Migrant workers, and Migrant workers as a proportion of all workers.

Source: ILO, 2018

Table 2.2 shows that over 111 million migrant workers, 68 per cent, were in the high-income countries with a sixth of the world's 3.5 billion workers. Migrants were almost 20 per cent of workers in high-income countries, but less than five per cent of workers in low-income countries.

By region, 24 per cent of migrant workers in 2017 were in Europe, 23 per cent were in North America, and 14 per cent were in the Arab states. Almost 41 per cent of all workers in the Arab states were migrants, followed by 21 per cent of all workers in North America and 18 per cent of all workers in Europe.

Covid-19 and Migrant Exceptions

Many governments ordered non-essential businesses to close in March 2020, and closed their borders to non-essential travelers as Covid-19 spread around the world. Agriculture was considered an essential industry by most governments, which means that farm and food system workers were expected to report to work despite general stay-at-home orders. Similarly, most governments made exceptions for truckers and others moving food and other items from farmers to supermarkets and over national borders (Moroz, Shrestha and Testaverde, 2020).

Food system workers include higher-than-average shares of migrant workers in occupations that range from farm worker to food preparation worker. Many migrant restaurant workers lost their jobs as non-essential businesses were ordered to close, but most farm workers kept their jobs as food production ramped up in spring 2020 in the Northern Hemisphere.

Most governments have special programs that allow farmers to employ foreign workers to fill seasonal jobs (Martin, 2016). Despite record-high unemployment rates, governments opened otherwise closed borders to seasonal farm workers, prompting farmers in some countries to charter planes to transport workers over closed borders as with German farmers who arranged charter flights for Romanian workers (Alderman, Eddy and Tsang, 2020).

Many governments tried to persuade local jobless workers to accept seasonal farm jobs. The results were mixed. British labour recruiter Concordia reported that only 10 percent of the 1,000 British workers who responded to the "Pick for Britain" campaign in April 2020 went to work on farms; the others cited the short duration of the job, difficulties getting from their homes to farms with jobs, and the need to care for children. Many British farmers said they preferred experienced Bulgarians and Romanians to jobless local workers (O'Carroll, 2020).

Germany similarly created a web site (https://www.daslandhilft.de/) to link jobless nonfarm workers with seasonal farm jobs, and provided economic incentives to do farm work. Furloughed workers who accepted farm jobs could continue to receive the 80 per cent of the regular pay paid to furloughed workers and work up to 115 days in a seasonal farm job without paying social security taxes on the farm earnings. However, most local workers did not start or stay in seasonal farm jobs (Eddy, 2020).

A million people are employed in Italian agriculture. In 2020, some 150,000 Eastern European migrants could not travel to Italy to fill farm jobs, prompting efforts to attract jobless Italians into farm work. Some farmers reported that five or more Italians applied for each seasonal job available, but that many of the Italians who started to do farm work soon quit. A $1.1 billion farm support proposal in May 2020 included legalization for unauthorized farm workers, which critics said would not add to the seasonal farm workforce since the unauthorized workers who would benefit were already in Italy (Horowitz, 2020).

Figure 2.1 shows that the US food system accounts for 11 per cent of US jobs, many of which are seasonal or part time and most of which are in sectors that process, sell, and serve consumers, including 60 per cent in food service and eating and drinking place. Hired workers account for 1.5 million or almost 60 per cent of average employment in farming. However, since many farm jobs are seasonal, some 2.5 million unique workers are employed sometime during the year for wages on US farms.

Most of the hired farm workers in the US were born in Mexico, and about half are not authorized to work in the US, which limits their access to government Covid-19 relief programs. There were fears that Covid-19 could spread rapidly among hired farm workers, many of whom live in crowded housing, but during the first three months of the pandemic there were few reports of farm workers contracting Covid-19 (Beatty et al., 2020). By contrast, there were well-publicized outbreaks of Covid-19 among meatpacking plants, which often employ refugees and other legal immigrant workers in (Groves and Tareen, 2020).

Meat and poultry processing employed an average 520,000 workers in 2018 for average weekly wages of $800, and larger meatpackers often had to raise wages and offer bonuses to persuade meatpacking workers to continue reporting to work.

Relatively few jobless US workers sought seasonal farm jobs in 2020 for several reasons. First, most jobless workers are in cities and lack links to the labour contractors and crew bosses who match most farm workers with jobs and housing in agricultural areas. Second, unemployment benefits may exceed agricultural earnings. A laid-off California worker who was earning $3,000 a month would receive $350 a week in unemployment benefits, plus $600 a week in federal pandemic unemployment benefits through July 31, 2020, making benefits of $950 a week more than the $500 a week average earnings of employees of labour contractors (Rural Migration News, 2020a).

Instead of hiring jobless workers in the US, more farm employers requested certification to employ H-2A foreign workers in 2020 (Rural Migration News, 2020b). The H-2A program allows farm employers to recruit and employ foreign workers to fill farm jobs that last up to 10 months. The US Department of Labor (DOL) certified 257,666 jobs to be filled with

H-2A workers in FY19, and the US Department of State (DOS) issued almost 205,000 H-2A visas, over 90 per cent to Mexicans (some H-2A visa holders fill two farm jobs while in the US).

Figure 2.1. Employment in the US Food System, 2018

Employment in agriculture, food, and related industries, 2018

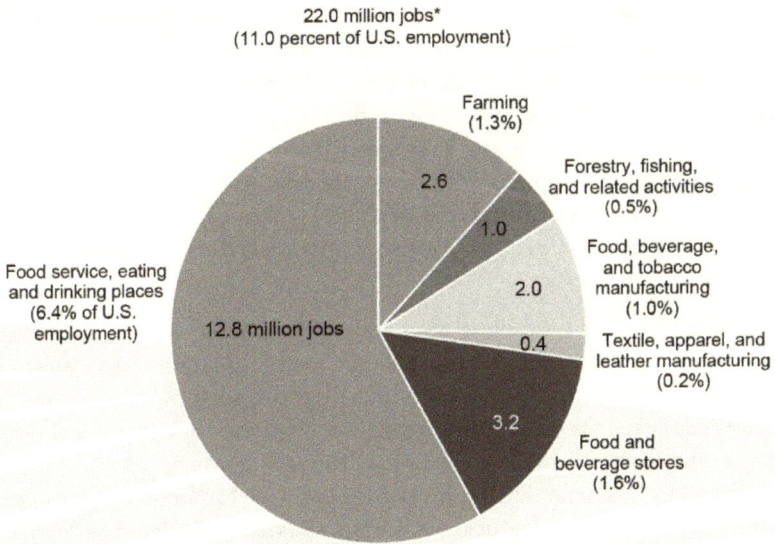

22.0 million jobs*
(11.0 percent of U.S. employment)

Farming
(1.3%)

2.6

Forestry, fishing,
and related activities
(0.5%)

1.0

Food, beverage,
and tobacco
manufacturing
(1.0%)

2.0

Food service, eating
and drinking places
(6.4% of U.S.
employment)

12.8 million jobs

0.4

Textile, apparel, and
leather manufacturing
(0.2%)

3.2

Food and
beverage stores
(1.6%)

*Full- and part-time jobs.

Source:https://www.ers.usda.gov/data-products/ag-and-food   statistics-charting-the-essentials/ag-and-food-sectors-and-the-economy/

The number of US farm jobs certified to be filled with H-2A workers remained below 100,000 until 2014, doubled to over 200,000 in 2017, and has continued to increase despite Covid-19. As part of the immigration exceptions for agriculture, the US DOS granted visas to H-2A workers without the in-person interviews that are normally required. Two-thirds of H-2A visas are issued in Monterrey, Mexico, where US consular officers issue up to 2,000 H-2A visas a day.

Conclusions

The Covid-19 pandemic is widely expected to transform labour markets, substituting machines for workers to reduce the risk of the virus. Even after stay-at-home orders are lifted, there are predictions of less employment in the food and beverage industry as take out and consumption at home replace restaurant meals and drinking in bars.

Agriculture has always been a slightly different industry, and was treated differently during the Covid-19 pandemic. Farming was considered an essential business, with farm workers expected to report to work. Governments that could not persuade jobless local workers to fill seasonal farm jobs instead made exceptions to closed borders for foreign farm workers.

The Covid-19 pandemic is likely to add to rising farm labour costs, which in turn will accelerate the three major labour trends in industrial country agriculture: labour-saving mechanization, more guest workers, and more imports of labour-intensive commodities. Mechanizing hand tasks on farms requires a systems perspective, cooperation between biologists and engineers, and trial-and-error innovation. This means examining the entire process from farm to fork, developing uniformly ripening commodities that can be harvested in one pass through the field, and perhaps separating machine and hand harvested commodities at supermarkets in a manner similar to conventional and organic.

The failure of local jobless workers to fill seasonal farm jobs during the pandemic has seemingly persuaded many governments that only international migrant workers will accept most seasonal farm jobs. Most governments require farm employers to try and fail to recruit local workers before they are allowed to employ foreign guest workers, but these recruitment efforts rarely find local workers. Governments require farmers to pay for their workers' housing and transportation, which raises farm labour costs but provides employers with reliable workers who will not abandon their jobs in the middle of the season.

Finally, the pandemic could increase trade in labour-intensive commodities. The virus is not spread via food and, with the same production technologies but lower labour costs in developing countries, more fresh fruits and vegetables could be produced in one country and consumed in another. The US already imports half of its fresh fruit, and a third of its fresh vegetables, most from Mexico, and the share of imports in fruit and vegetable consumption is rising (Escobar, Martin, and Starbridis, 2019).

Covid-19 introduces new uncertainties for everyone. For agriculture, the longer term effects of the pandemic include faster mechanization, more guest workers, and rising imports. Responses are likely to vary by commodity and be shaped by government policies. For example, if governments subsidize mechanization and open their borders to fresh produce, there are likely to be fewer guest workers. Alternatively, easing farmer access to guest workers and closing borders to imported produce means more international migrant workers.

References

Alderman, L., M. Eddy and A. Tsang (2020). Migrant Farmworkers Whose Harvests Feed Europe Are Blocked at Borders. New York Times. March 27. https://www.nytimes.com/2020/03/27/business/coronavirus-farm-labor-europe.html?searchResultPosition=1

Beatty, T., A. Hill, P. Martin, and Z. Rutledge (2020). COVID-19 and Farm Workers: Challenges Facing California Agriculture. ARE Update. Vol 23. No 5. https://giannini.ucop.edu/publications/are-update/issues/2020/23/5/ covid-19-and-farm-workers-challenges-facing-califo/

Eddy, M. (2020). Farm Workers Airlifted Into Germany Provide Solutions and Pose New Risks. May 18. New York Times. https://www.nytimes.com/2020/05/18/world/europe/coronavirus-german-farms-migrant-workers-airlift.html

Escobar, A., P. Martin, O. Starbridis (2019). Farm Labor and Mexico's Export Produce Industry. Wilson Center. www.wilsoncenter.org/publication/farm-labor-and-mexicos-export-produce-industry

Groves, S. and S. Tareen (2020). Worker shortage concerns loom in immigrant-heavy meatpacking. Washington Post. https://www.washingtonpost.com/business/worker-shortage-concerns-loom-in-immigrant-heavy-meatpacking/2020/05/25/0ebb5bde-9f02-11ea-be06-af5514ee0385_story.html

Horowitz, J. (2020). For Some Italians, the Future of Work Looks Like the Past. New York Times. https://www.nytimes.com/2020/05/24/world/europe/italy-farms-coronavirus.html?searchResultPosition=1

ILO (2020). Protecting migrant workers during the COVID-19 pandemic. https://www.ilo.org/global/topics/labour-migration/publications/WCMS_743268/lang--en/index.htm

ILO (2018). Global Estimates on International Migrant Workers – Results and Methodology. www.ilo.org/global/about-the-ilo/newsroom/news/WCMS_652106/lang--en/index.htm

Martin, P. (2016). Migrant Workers in Commercial Agriculture. ILO. http://www.ilo.org/global/topics/labour-migration/publications/WCMS_538710/lang--en/index.htm

Moroz, H., M. Shrestha and M. Testaverde (2020). Potential Responses to the COVID-19 Outbreak in Support of Migrant Workers. World Bank. https://elibrary.worldbank.org/doi/abs/10.1596/33625

O'Carroll, L. (2020). British workers reject fruit-picking jobs as Romanians flown in. Guardian. April 17. https://www.theguardian.com/environment/2020/apr/17/british-workers-reject-fruit-picking-jobs-as-romanians-flown-in-coronavirus

Rural Migration News (2020a). Labor, Virus, H-1B. Vol 26. No 2. https://migration.ucdavis.edu/rmn/more.php?id=2413

Rural Migration News (2020b). H-2A, H-2B. Vol 26. No 2. https://migration.ucdavis.edu/rmn/more.php?id=2420.

CHAPTER 3

HOSTAGES OF MOBILITY: TRANSPORT, SECURITIZATION AND STRESS DURING PANDEMIC[1]

Biao Xiang

Part One:

Historically, epidemics have been closely related to population mobility. The COVID-19 outbreak is special in that, population mobility in China in the year 2020 is not only unprecedentedly prevalent and frequent, but has also become a prerequisite for the economy and many people's livelihoods. The circulation of goods and the movement of people are arguably more important than assembly lines in factories in sustaining economic growth. The COVID-19 epidemic and the subsequent responses are particularly impactful because they abruptly halt what we may call a "mobility economy".

This specific context can be discerned through a comparison to the severe acute respiratory syndrome (SARS) outbreak in 2003. Striving to contain the SARS virus, the Chinese government singled out rural-urban migrants as the priority target. At least 8 urgent directives about migrants were issued by the central government and 16 by Beijing municipality government in April and May 2003. In 2020, however, migrant workers are hardly mentioned. Most measures fighting COVID-19 target the entire population. It is clear that mobility is no longer specific to migrants and has become a generalized feature across society. The meaning of mobility has changed, as has its relation to public health. There were good reasons why the government targeted migrants in 2003. Rural-urban migrants contributed 14.81 percent of all SARS cases in the peak of the epidemic (Ministry of Health, 2003). An estimated 12.6% of all migrants nationwide left cities in the wake of the outbreak (Agriculture Survey Team, National Bureau of Statistics, cited in Ma

---

[1] This chapter comprises three research blog essays previously published in the COMPAS Coronavirus and Mobility Forum facilitated by Biao Xiang: Part 1: https://www.compas.ox.ac.uk/ 2020/from-chain-reaction-to-grid-reaction-mobilitiesrestrictions-during-sars-coronavirus/ on 12/03/2020. Part 2: https://www.compas.ox.ac.uk/2020/point-to-point-labour-transport-the-post-lockdown-securitization-of-mobility/ 22/04/2020. Part 3: https://www.compas.ox.ac.uk/2020/mobile-livelihoods-in-stress/ on 26/03/2020 .

2003) and they became the main source of rural infections. A Beijing Academy of Social Sciences researcher commented that "the spread of the epidemic caused by the fleeing of migrants from Beijing due to the outbreak, and the explosive growth of SARS cases inside of Beijing caused by the concentration of migrants, for the first time brings migrants' health issue to public attention in an extremely extraordinarily way." (Feng, 2003: 10).

Chain reactions

How exactly was the SARS epidemic related to population mobility? My fieldwork at that time suggests that, despite narratives in public media and policy documents, few migrants left the city because of health concerns. Migrants were much less sensitive to the epidemic threat than their urban middle-class counterparts. Migrants' mobility was a result of a chain reaction. In late April 2003, after two months' cover up, and under strong pressure from the international community and domestic urban residents, the Chinese government acknowledged the epidemic as a national emergency. Public entertainment venues and construction sites were considered high-risk areas and were shut down overnight. Beijing closed about 70 percent of all restaurants in May (Yang, 2003), which put up to 237,300 migrants' jobs in jeopardy (my estimate based on Xinhua News Agency, 2003). Jobless, migrants had to go home. They became the worst victims of the virus, of economic disruption, and of social stigma. Chain reaction means that the connection between epidemic and migration was mediated by social stratification (Xiang, 2003).

Grid reactions

In comparison, the COVID-19 epidemic has triggered grid reactions. Residential communities, districts, cities and even entire provinces act as grids to impose blanket surveillance over all the residents, minimize mobilities, and isolate themselves. In the Chinese administrative system, a grid is a cluster of households, ranging from 50 in the countryside to 1000 in cities. Grid managers (normally volunteers) and grid heads (cadres who receive state salaries) make sure that rubbish is collected on time, cars are parked properly, and no political demonstration is possible. During the outbreak, grid managers visit door to door to check everyone's temperature, hand out passes which allow one person per household to leave home twice a week and, in the case of collective quarantine, deliver food to the doorstep of all families three times a day. A grid reaction, just like the COVID-19 virus itself, is highly contagious. Once the central government declared the war on the virus, localities across the nation adopted strict measures, even in remote places with no reported infection. In no time the entire nation put itself under gridlock. Grid reaction is not about community grids only; it refers to an all-out, undifferentiated, war-like strategy. Turning entire hospitals into COVID wards and building barricades around villages are part of the grid reaction too.

Hyper-mobility

Total (im)mobilization is regarded necessary partly because of unprecedented mobility levels in China. Over 3.6 billion Chinese travelled by train and 660 million by air in 2019, compared to 0.95 billion and 87 million respectively in 2003; the number of private motor vehicles increased from 13 million in 2003 to 206 million (CEIC Data, 2020). Mobility has increased also because job is casualized. Between 2008 and 2016, the informal sector generated 10 million jobs a year, while stable employment in state owned enterprises and foreign-owned enterprises increased much slower and in fact shrank by nearly 2 million between 2015 and 2016 (Qian, 2020: 2). The labor dispatch service was legalized in 2008, which by 2011 accounted for 13.1% of all the jobs nationwide (National Federation of Trade Unions, 2012: 35). Dispatch agencies move workers from one project site to another. Many others apart from rural-urban migrants are now moving between places and between jobs. This also means that government can no longer rely on employers as a mediator in monitoring employees. Feasible measures have to target the population in entirety. Grid reaction can be deeply disruptive Firstly, just like chain reaction, grid reaction induced unintended movements that may further spread the virus. The Wuhan lock down triggered flights from the city, which is said to have turned Wenzhou into an epicentre outside of Hubei (Yao, 2020). Inside Hubei, the shortage of medical resources resulting from the lock down compelled patients to move from hospital to hospital seeking care, often on foot because of the suspension of transport. As grids are based on physical boundaries, grid reaction has also fuelled alarming place-based stigma. Persons originally from infected places, regardless how long they had been away, were locked in at home by neighbours, and were even attacked online. Reports also show rising conflicts between residents and officials due to forced quarantine.

Disruptions in economy are the most obvious. As China's economy in 2020 is four times that of its 2003 size, and, more importantly, as it plays a central role in global supply chains, any glitch in circulation has far-reaching consequences. But it must be emphasized that those who rely on mobility for their livelihood may suffer the most. Taxi drivers, delivery workers, staff in the logistics and service sectors cannot work without moving, and will have no customers without others on the move. Many of them live on daily wages. Two months' standing still could be devastating. Thus a Catch-22 scenario: prevalent mobility leaves the government with few options other than grid reaction, but it at the same time renders such response unbearably disruptive. When Chinese society becomes more mobile, responses to risks appear more crude and clumsy. How can a mobility economy be organized in a more sustainable and equitable matter? This is a fundamental challenge for researchers and policy makers in coming decades.

Part Two: Point-to-point labour transport: the post-lockdown securitization of mobility

"Point-to-point" labour transport has become the standard way in which China is resuming labour mobility during the easing of lockdown. Since 8 February 2020, the central government has urged employers and local governments to bring the 170 million rural-urban migrants, the majority of whom went home for the Chinese New Year in January and were subsequently confined in the countryside, back to work. This is done in a "point A-to-point B" manner: migrants are transported from home to the workplace directly in groups, led by designated personnel, on designated vehicles, following designated routes, to the designated enterprise. Each bus should be no more than half-full to allow for social distancing, and the last two rows are reserved as an isolation area in case passengers develop fever. Each migrant must go through a health check before departure, and have their temperature checked throughout the journey. All the migrants' information, compiled and updated by the designated organizer, must be handed over to the employer on arrival.

In this way, more than 5 million migrants were transported on 200,000 charted coaches and 367 charted trains between mid-February and the end of March (People's Daily, 2020). This happens outside China too. Thousands of agricultural workers have been airlifted from Eastern Europe to Germany and the UK, and from Mexico to Canada, since early April. Mobility as an economic necessity and as a security concern "Point-to-point" is precisely how I have characterized unskilled labour migration from China to Japan, South Korea and Singapore since the early 2000s. The transnational migrants "are extracted from their hometowns and inserted in a foreign workplace…migration in this case is not about how migrants move and explore, but is about how they are moved with great precision." The control of labour in the worksite is supplemented, or even substituted, by the control of transnational mobility. For instance, when labour disputes arise, enterprises and labour intermediaries would send the worker back to China as a way to "settle" the case, which effectively discipline workers in their daily activity. Migrant workers are regulated more as mobile subjects than as workers.

During the current pandemic, the double pressure of containing the virus and of reviving the economy renders mobility a necessity and a security concern. The securitization of mobility means that (1) mundane mobility is associated with existential threats to the collective; (2) surveillance is imposed on all in order to prevent exceptions. Proportionality is out of the window: a single terrorist attack, or a single infection case, is regarded too many; (3) normal rules are suspended and extraordinary measures are introduced (Buzan et al., 1998). The securitization of international migration is not new, as widely documented in border studies. However, point-to-point transport is not concerned with who the foreigner is or what he/she wants to do, but instead focuses on how a person, in most cases a perfectly legitimate citizen, moves physically in a way that would not undermine health security. Borders appear irrelevant. The emphasis is to "tunnel" (Graham and Marvin, 2001) labour from one point to another directly, bypassing the space between, including all the borders.

Government and platforms

The distinction between "human security" and "state security" has collapsed in the pandemic. The role of the Chinese government is central in point-to-point transport. Provincial governments, in both labour-sending and -receiving places, take charge of overall planning, prefecture governments identify demands and supplies, according to which counties of the sending place monitor the transport to eliminate gaps between "the home gate, the bus gate, and the factory gate."(Jianhua, 2020). The Ministry of Transport has set up emergency telephone lines in its Logistics Security Office to deal with incidents during the transport (Ministry of Transport, 2020). Provincial and prefectural governments on the receiving side are the main funded of this operation. They pay for the transport and even hand out cash to migrant workers on arrival. The Chinese government also set up multiple on-line platforms to securitize labour mobility. The Platform for Rural-Urban Migrants Returning to Work, launched by the Ministry of Human Resources and Social Security, enables governments and enterprises to coordinate in arranging transport. The National Road Passenger Service Management Platform, managed by the Ministry of Transport, collects detailed travel plans to make sure that the feeder stations on the way will carry out health checks and provide food and water without delay. There are also platforms and apps for enterprises or migrants to seek help (Ying, 2020). Real-time Health QR Code generated by mobile phones, which shows whether the individual has COVID symptoms and whether contacted possible infection sources in the past 14 days, is checked all the time. This Code is necessary for boarding a local bus or even, in many cities, stepping out of one's gated community. Intermediaries: securitization of mobility + casualization of work?

Clearly, the Government may not carry out point-to-point labour transport for long. But other actors may use this as an opportunity to flourish. Commercial labour intermediaries, ranging from individual gangmasters to large labour dispatchment corporations, are explicitly encouraged by the government in the resumption of mobility. Guangdong province in south China promises to reward an intermediary US$25 for recruiting a worker, and US$700 for organizing an online job fair that attracts over 300 corporate participants. Intermediaries that specialize in domestic helpers are singled out as a priority for support: high-performing agencies are given one-time grants of US$30,000-40,000 each (Guangdong Provincial Government, 2020). In addition to recruiting and managing a flexible labour force, intermediaries are now organizing labour mobility. As mobility becomes a security concern, organizing mobility becomes a new business niche. Domestic workers agencies—estimated to be 750,000 strong nationwide in 2020—receive special support since the securitization of domestic workers' mobility is regarded particularly important in the battle against the virus. As intermediaries gain an even stronger footing, the securitization of mobility may become the other side of the deepening casualization of work.

Part Three: Mobile Livelihoods in Stress

The COVID-19 pandemic reminds us of just how many people across the world rely on mobility for their livelihood: taxi drivers, delivery workers, street vendors, maintenance technicians of long-distance operation systems, all employees in the hospitality sector… not forgetting the most vulnerable at this time, the homeless, beggars and street kids, especially in the global South, who have to move from place to place to get food, to find a place to sleep through the night, and to run away from police. People with mobile livelihoods are not the same as migrant workers. They bear a number of distinctive features:

• mobility is their main means of work, rather than simply a way to access jobs as in the case of migrant workers;

• they rely on others' mobilities to create demands for their work;

• increasingly commonly, they work in precarious conditions without long-term security, which partly explains why

• they not only move between places, but also between jobs frequently;

• through constant movement they seek higher pay and cope with various problems such as work disputes or family needs. Mobility is a source of vulnerability, but is also a coping method. Immobility deprives them of their basic coping resource and thus exacerbates vulnerability;

• their work, delivered on the move, tends to be immaterial, non-accumulative and extremely time-sensitive.

While manufacturers can make up for lost time by extra work later, service workers cannot reverse the loss of economic opportunities. For them the loss is like the loss of time itself. If a taxi driver can't work for a month, he/she can't expect the number of customers in the next month would double the usual. There is no such thing as "delay" in mobile livelihoods.

"Work from home" is now a requirement, but not everyone can afford to do so. Immobility is a privilege, and self isolation a luxury. For many, staying at home simply means being jobless. A mobile livelihood is more than mobile work The prevalence of mobile livelihoods, in both the global North and South, is clearly associated with structural changes in the economy. But individuals' choice matters too. According to a survey by Meituan, the largest food delivery company in China, 64.0% of its riders identified "time flexibility" as the most important reason why they chose the job, by far the most popular reason. 58.8% of riders work less than 4 hours a day on delivery; multitasking is the normal working life for them (Meituan Research Institute, 2020). Driving taxis for app companies appeals to young people partly because the job is associated with car ownership, a typical symbol of the middle class. Mobility is thus a livelihood strategy, namely how "people pursue a range of livelihood outcomes (health, income, reduced vulnerability, etc.) by drawing on a range of assets to pursue a variety of activities. The activities they adopt and the way they reinvest in asset building are driven in part by their own preferences and priorities." (Farrington, 1999). In order to understand mobile livelihoods, we need to know what the actors do, what they have, as well as what they desire and what they avoid.

Mobility assemblages

Not all people with mobile livelihoods are affected by the shutdowns in the same way. In China for instance, truck drivers, taxi drivers and delivery riders have experienced the epidemic differently. Truck drivers have been affected severely. According to a nation-wide survey on 23 February, one month after the Wuhan lock down, 75.4% of the surveyed truck drivers could not work at all since the virus outbreak; 90% of them reported to feel "extreme" or "considerable" economic stress. They identified vehicle loans and house mortgage as the two main sources of the hardship (Chuanhua Charity Foundation Public Welfare Institute, 2020). In contrast, food delivery riders witnessed surge of job opportunities. Between 20 January and 18 March 2020, Meituan alone recruited 336,000 riders, in addition to the 4 million in 2019. More than 60% of the new recruits had lost jobs in manufacturing or service due to the shutdown (Meituan Research Institute, 2020).

Taxi drivers' experiences are more differentiated. Orders of taxis (including on-line hailing riding) dropped by 85% in February (Ministry of Transport, 2020). Some drivers lost up to 80% of incomes in the worst week even though they were outside the epicentre, others suffered less. This depended on which financial scheme the driver chose when signing contracts with the car rental company (Xiaobin, 2020). Thus, mobilities are mobility assemblages—mixes of different types of mobilities. The halt of population movement can be more accurately understood as a redistribution of mobilities: empty trains are accompanied by the intensified movements of "key workers". Mobility assemblages are also manifested by long-distance truck drivers shifting to short-distance transport, and hotel staff becoming delivery workers. We need to examine the relations between different modes of mobilities and the dynamics of how mobile livelihoods mutate.

The future for mobile livelihoods

The fact that 336,000 workers in China lost their regular jobs and became Meituan riders may indicate that mobile livelihoods will become even more prevalent in the future. Another curious development is that, despite the acute need for timely goods delivery, truck drivers reported a minimum of 20% drop in their renumeration, and the trend continued after the transport restriction was lifted. Could it be that app companies are taking a bigger share of profits in a time when the total revenue shrank? This is what makes mobile livelihoods in the 21st century so different from their historical predecessors such as itinerant merchants, seasonal agricultural workers, and peasant "target earners" (Piore, 1979). Mobile livelihoods today are intensively mediated through large digital platforms and complicated financial packages. For instance car rental companies in China turned online hailing rides into a range of financial packages to be sold to the drivers, which mitigated the impacts of the disruption on some drivers but exacerbated for others. Thinking of our post-pandemic life, we should think not only whether we need more or less mobility, but also how mobile livelihoods should be organized.

References

Buzan, B., Wæver, O. and de Wilde, J. (1998). Security: A New Framework for Analysis. Boulder, CO: Lynne Rienner.

CEIC Data. 2020. "China: Transport and Telecommunication", https://www.ceicdata.com/en/country/china. Accessed on 25 February 2020.

Chuanhua Charity Foundation Public Welfare Institute (2020). 2020 Survey on Chinese truck drivers. https://www.thepaper.cn/newsDetail_forward_6435075

Farrington, J., D. Carney, C. Ashley and C. Turton (1999). Sustainable Livelihoods in Practice. Early Applications of Concepts in Rural Areas. Natural Resources Perspectives 42. London: Overseas Development Institute.

Feng Xiaoying. 2003. Feidian yu liudong renkou guanli moshi gaige lujing de xuanze (SARS and the Choice of Reform Paths for Migrant Population Management Model). Chengshi Wenti (Urban Issues). 4 (114): 9-12.

Graham, S. and Marvin, S. (2001). Splintering Urbanism: Networked Infrastructures, Technological Mobilities, and the Urban Condition. London and New York: Routledge.

Guangdong Provincial Government (2020, 20 February). "Several Policy Measures to Stabilize and Promote Employment in Guangdong Province" http://www.gz.gov.cn/xw/jrgz/content/post_5731279.html

Jianhua, S. (2020). Deputy Director, Poverty Alleviation Office of Ministry of Human Resources and Social Security, 7 March 2020, presentation at State Council press conference on the work of guaranteeing "point-to-point" service for the return of migrant workers, http://www.mot.gov.cn/2020wangshangzhibo/yqfk9/)

Ma Xiaohe. 2003. Jiji caiqu youxiao cuoshi fangzhi feidian zaocheng nongmin shouru xiahua (Take Proactive Measures to Prevent Farmers' Income Loss). In Research Report Series of Macro Economic Research Academy, Economic Development Committee of China, 9 June. Available at http://www.amr.gov.cn/macro_economic/index.jsp?subframeid=1 , accessed on 6 January 2004.

Meituan Research Institute (2020-03-19). Report on Meituan riders' employment during the 2019-2020 epidemic. https://www.sohu.com/a/381389256_115402 4

Ministry of Health, China. "Quezhen binli an zhiye fenbu" (Distribution of confirmed cases by occupation). In Chuanranxing Feidianxing Feiyan Yiqing Dili Xinxi Xitong (Geographic Information System on Infectious Atypical Pneumonia). Available at http:168.160.224.167/sarsmap, accessed on 16 July 2003

Ministry of Transport (2020). "Notice on Guaranteeing Transport Service for Migrant Workers' Return to Work" Code: 2020-03068, Transport [2020] No. 56, February 11, 2020; http://xxgk.mot.gov.cn/jigou/ysfws/202002/t20200211_3331884.html

Ministry of Transport (2020, 10 March). Orders for taxis dropped by 85% in February. No.1 Finance and Economy. https://www.yicai.com/brief/100536579.html

National Federation of Trade Unions Research Team on Labor Dispatch, 2012, Dangqian woguo laowu paiqian yonggong dizwei diaocha. [A survey on the current employment status of labor dispatch in China], Zhongguo Laodong [China Labor], No. 5: 23.

People's Daily (2020). "Let migrant workers return to work smoothly and do their jobs contently" 13 April 2020 http://society.people.com.cn/n1/2020/0413/c1008-31670439.html

Piore, M. (1979). Birds of Passage: Migrant Labour and Industrial Societies. Cambridge University Press.

Qian Jiwei. 2020. Under-coverage of Social Insurance in China's Informal Economy. No. 9. EAI Commentary. https://research.nus.edu.sg/eai/ wpcontent/uploads/sites/2/2020/02/EAIC-09-20200203.pdf

Xiang, Biao. 2003. SARS and Migrant Workers in China. Asian and Pacific Migration Journal. 12 (4): 467-499.

Xiaobin, K. (2020). Online ride-hailing in the shadow of the epidemic: some drivers' income plunges 80%. February 11. Interface News. https://cj.sina.com.cn/articles/view/3243067320/c14d47b801900n8q6

Xinhua News Agency. 2003. "Diaocha xianshi: zhonggou yin feidian fanxiang nongming bacheng reng zai dengdai guangwang" (Survey shows 80 per cent of returned migrants due to Atypical Pneumonia still wait and see), 19 June.

Yang Bin. 2003. Feidian kenan daozhi Beijing canyinye 5000 jia chuju (Atypical Pneumonia may force 5,000 restaurants out of business), Sinanews, 4 June.

Yao, Gaoyuan (Mayor of Wenzhou), Zhejiang province, Interview at China Central TV News 1 + 1 column, 2 February 2020. Available on https://www.youtube.com/watch?v=aHh2jiScjIE.

Ying, Z. (2020). Director, Employment Promotion Department, Ministry of Human Resources and Social Security, 7 March 2020, presentation at State Council press conference, ibid.

CHAPTER 4

MODELING AND PREDICTION OF THE 2019 CORONAVIRUS DISEASE SPREADING IN CHINA INCORPORATING HUMAN MIGRATION DATA

Choujun Zhan, Chi Kong Tse, Yuxia Fu, Zhikang Lai, Haijun Zhang

Introduction

The Novel Coronavirus Disease 2019 (COVID-19) began to spread since December 2019 from Wuhan, a centrally located city in China with a population of 11 million, to almost all provinces throughout China and 213 other countries. On February 19, 2020 (when this work was completed), a total of 74,579 cases of COVID-19 infection were confirmed in China, and the death toll reached 2,119. Moreover, as human-to-human transmission had been found to occur in some early Wuhan cases in mid-December (Li et al., 2020), the high volume and frequency of movement of people from Wuhan to other cities and between cities was an obvious cause for the wide and rapid spread of the disease throughout the country. Prior study also suggested strong correlation between the spreading of infectious diseases with intercity travel (Colizza et al., 2006). The Susceptible-Exposed-Infected-Removed (SEIR) model has traditionally been used to study epidemic spreading with various forms of networks of transmission which define the contact topology (Diekmann, Heesterbeek & Britton, 2013), such as scalefree networks (Pastor et al., 2001; Boguna et al., 2003; Small & Tse, 2006), small-world networks (Small & Tse, 2005), Oregon graph (Wang et al., 2003; Chakrabarti et al., 2008), and adaptive networks (Gross, D'Lima & Blasius, 2006). Moreover, in most studies, the contact process assumed that the contagion expanded at a certain rate from an infected individual to his/her neighbour, and that the spreading process took place in a single population (network).

The COVID-19 outbreak, however, began to occur and escalated in a special holiday period in China (about 20 days surrounding the Lunar New Year), during which a huge volume of intercity travel took place, resulting in outbreaks in multiple regions connected by an active transportation network. Thus, in order to understand the COVID-19 spreading process in China, it is essential to examine the human migration dynamics, especially between the epicentre Wuhan and other Chinese cities. Recent studies have also revealed the risk of transmission of the virus from Wuhan to other cities (Du et al., 2020), and such risk was found to be realistic.

In this chapter, we utilise the human migration data collected from Baidu Migration (2020), which provides historical indicative daily volume of travellers to/from and between 367 cities in China. To demonstrate the impact of intercity traffic on the COVID-19 epidemic spreading, we plot in Figure 4.1 the number of infected individuals in different cities versus the inflow traffic volume from Wuhan, which clearly shows that for cities farther away from Wuhan, the number of infected individuals almost increases linearly with the inflow traffic from Wuhan. In view of the importance of human migration dynamics to the disease spreading process, we combine, in this study, intercity travel data collected from Baidu Migration (2020) with the traditional SEIR model (Diekmann, Heesterbeek & Britton, 2013) to build a new dynamic transmission model for the spreading of COVID-19 in China.

Figure 4.1. Number of infected individuals in various cities on February 13, 2020 versus the city's inflow traffic from Wuhan. Inflow traffic of each city from Wuhan is quantified by migration strength from Wuhan extracted from Baidu Migration data.

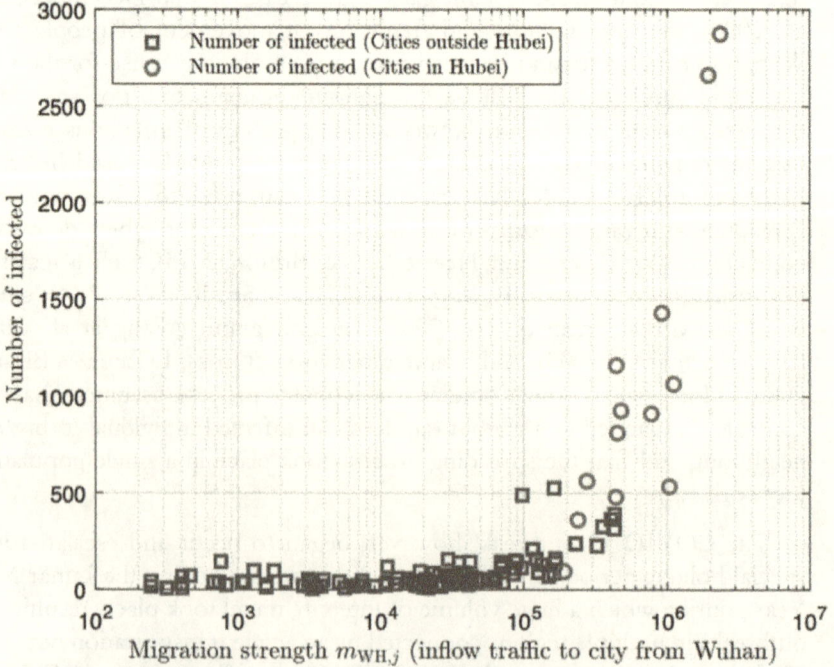

Using official historical data of infected, recovered and death cases in 367 cities, we performed fitting of the data to estimate the best set of model parameters, which were then used to estimate the number of individuals exposed to the virus in each city and to predict the extent of spreading in the coming months. We predicted on February 18, 2020, that provided such migration control and other stringent measures continued to be in place, the number of infected cases in various Chinese cities would peak between late February to early March 2020, with about 0.8%, less than 0.1% and less than 0.01% of the population eventually infected in Wuhan, Hubei Province, and the rest of China, respectively. Moreover, for most cities in and outside Hubei Province (except Wuhan), the total number of infected individuals would be less than 4000 and 300, respectively. Finally, as the effectiveness of treatment improved, the recovery rate would increase and the epidemic was expected to end by June 2020.

Figure 4.2. Daily data of COVID-19 infections in six Chinese cities from December 8, 2019 to February 13, 2020. (a) Wuhan (available from December 8, 2019); (b) Beijing (available from January 20, 2020); (c) Chongqing (available from January 20, 2020); (d) Shenzhen (available from January 19, 2020); (e) Guangzhou (available from January 21, 2020); (d) Tianjin (available from January 21, 2020).

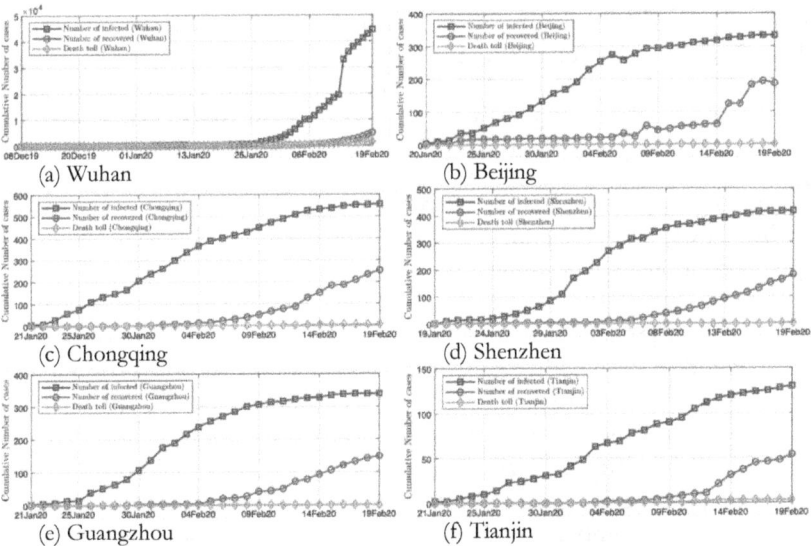

(a) Wuhan   (b) Beijing   (c) Chongqing   (d) Shenzhen   (e) Guangzhou   (f) Tianjin

In the remainder of the chapter, we first introduce the official daily infection data and the intercity migration data used in this study. The SEIR model is modified to incorporate the human migration dynamics, giving a realistic model suitable for studying the COVID-19 epidemic spreading dynamics. Historical data of infected, recovered and death cases from official source and data of daily intercity traffic (number of travellers between cities) extracted from Baidu Migration were used to generate the model parameters, which then enabled estimation of the propagation of the epidemic in the coming months. We will conclude with a brief interpretation of our estimation of the propagation and the reasonableness of our estimation in view of the measures taken by the Chinese authorities in controlling the spreading of this new disease.

Data Sources and Handling

The availability of official data of infected cases in China varies from city to city. Wuhan, being the epicentre, has the first confirmed case of COVID-19 infection on December 8, 2019 (Li et al., 2020). Most other cities in China began to report cases of COVID-19 infections around mid-January 2020. Our data of daily infected and recovered cases, and death tolls, were based on the official data released by the National Health Commission of China, and the daily data used in the prediction presented in this chapter were from January 24, 2020, to February 16, 2020, including the daily total number of confirmed cases in each city, daily total cumulative number of confirmed cases in each city, daily cumulative number of recovered cases in each city, and daily cumulative death toll in each city. It should be emphasised that the official data may not be the actual (true) data. Although the earliest confirmed case appeared on December 8, 2019, subsequent missing cases were expected to be significant in Hubei Province in the early stage of the epidemic outbreak. Systematic updates of infection data in other cities began after January 17, 2020. Figure 4.2 shows the number of confirmed infected cases, recovered cases and death tolls of six major Chinese cities.

As human-to-human transmission had been confirmed to occur in the spreading of COVID-19, gatherings of people and intercity travel of infected and exposed individuals within China were the main drives that escalated the spreading of the virus. The period (around 20 days) surrounding the Lunar New Year (mid-January to early February in 2020) was the most important holiday period in China. Migrant workers and students travelled from major cities to country towns for family reunion, and returned to the cities at the end of the holiday period. Holiday goers also travelled to and from tourist cities. China's Ministry of Transport estimated around 3 billion trips to be taken during this period each year. Wuhan, being a major transport hub and having a large number of higher education institutions as well as manufacturing plants, was among the cities with the largest outflow and inflow traffic before and after the Chinese New Year festival. Our study aims to incorporate these important human migration dynamics in the construction of the spreading model. We collected daily intercity travel data in China from Baidu Migration, which is a mobile app based big data system recording movements of mobile phone users. Specifically, we collected Baidu Migration data for 367 cities (or administrative regions) in China over the period of January 1, 2020, to February 13, 2020 in this study. The data provided the migration strengths of cities which were indicative measures of the human traffic volume moving in and out of individual cities and administrative regions. Based on the collected data, we construct the migration matrix, which is given as

$$
M(t) = \begin{bmatrix} m_{11}(t) & m_{12}(t) & \cdots & m_{1K}(t) \\ m_{21}(t) & m_{22}(t) & \cdots & m_{2K}(t) \\ \vdots & \vdots & \ddots & \vdots \\ m_{N1}(t) & m_{N2}(t) & \cdots & m_{KK}(t) \end{bmatrix} \tag{1}
$$

where K is the number of the cities or administrative regions (K = 367 in this study), and mij(t) is the migrant volume from city i to city j at time t. Migration matrix M thus effectively describes the network of cities with human movement constituting the links of the network. Several properties of M are worth noting:

M records migration from one city to another. Movement within a city is not counted, i.e., mii(t) = 0 for all i.

M is non-symmetric as traffic from one city to another is not necessarily reciprocal at any given time, i.e., mij(t) ≠ mji(t).

Number of outflow migrants of city i at time t is

$$
m_i^{(\text{out})}(t) = \sum_{i=j}^{K} m_{ij}(t). \tag{2}
$$

Number of inflow migrants of city i at time t is

$$
m_i^{(\text{in})}(t) = \sum_{j=1}^{K} m_{ji}(t). \tag{3}
$$

Figure 4.3. plots the daily total inflow and outflow migration strengths of Wuhan, showing the abrupt decrease of migration strengths after the city shut down all inbound and outbound traffic from January 24, 2020.

Figure 4.3. Total inflow/outflow of travellers to/from Wuhan from/to other Chinese cities using Baidu Migration data.

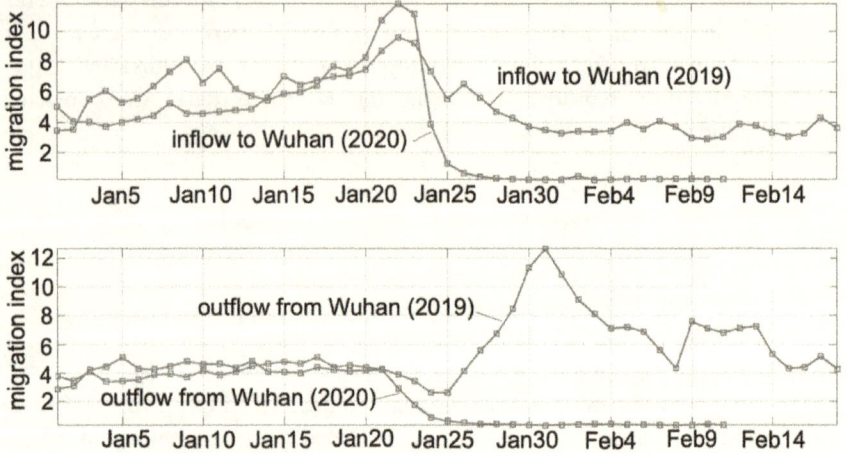

Methods of Modelling and Prediction

In the SEIR model, each individual in a population may assume one of four possible states at any time in the dynamic process of epidemic spreading, namely, susceptible (S), exposed (E), infected (I) and recovered/removed (R). The dynamics of the epidemic can be described by the following set of equations:

$$
\begin{cases}
\dot{S}(t) = -\beta S(t)I(t) \\
\dot{E}(t) = \beta S(t)I(t) - kE(t) \\
\dot{I}(t) = \kappa E(t) - \gamma I(t) \\
\dot{R}(t) = \gamma I(t)
\end{cases}
\tag{4}
$$

where S(t), E(t), I(t) and R(t) are, respectively, the number of people susceptible to the disease, exposed (being able to infect others but having no symptoms), infected (diagnosed as confirmed cases), and recovered (including death cases); β is the exposition rate (infection rate of susceptible individuals); k is the infection rate of exposed individuals; and g is the recovery rate. For simplicity, recovered individuals include patients recovered from the disease and death tolls. In discrete form, the SEIR model can be represented by

$$
\begin{aligned}
\Delta S(t) &= -\beta S(t-1)I(t-1), \\
\Delta E(t) &= \beta S(t-1)I(t-1) - \kappa E(t-1), \\
\Delta I(t) &= \kappa E(t-1) - \gamma I(t-1), \\
\Delta R(t) &= \gamma I(t-1)
\end{aligned}
\tag{5}
$$

where $\Delta S(t) = S(t)-S(t-1)$, $\Delta E(t) = E(t)-E(t-1)$, $\Delta I(t) = I(t)-I(t-1)$, and $\Delta R(t) = R(t)-R(t-1)$, with t being a daily count. As the incubation period for COVID-19 can be up to 14 days, the number of exposed individuals (who showed no symptom but were able to infect others) played a crucial role in the spreading of the disease. The state E, which is not available from the official data, is thus an important state in our model. Furthermore, combining death toll with the recovered number as state R will simplify the computation without affecting the accuracy of our data fitting and subsequent estimation.

Model

Suppose, for city i, the four states are Si(t), Ei(t), Ii(t) and Ri(t), at time t. Here, we also define a total susceptible population, N_i^s, which is the eventual number of infected individuals in city i. Moreover, if city i has a population of Pi and the eventual percentage of infection is di, then Nis = di Pi. Thus, we have

$$N_i^s(t) = S_i(t) + E_i(t) + I_i(t) + R_i(t). \quad (6)$$

The classic SEIR model would give $\Delta I(t)$ as the difference between the number of exposed individuals who become infected and the number of removed individuals. However, the onset of the COVID-19 epidemic had occurred in a special period of time in China, during which a huge migration traffic was being carried among cities, leading to a highly rapid transmission of the disease throughout the country. In view of this special migration factor, the SEIR model should incorporate the human migration dynamics in order to capture the essential features of the dynamics of the spreading. In particular, for city i, in addition to the abovementioned classic interpretation, the daily increase in the number of infected cases should also include the inflow of infected individuals from other cities, less the outflow of removed cases from city i. In reality, inflow and outflow of exposed individuals to and from the city are also important and to be estimated in the model. Thus, if mij(t) people move from city i to city j on day t, and the population of city i is Pi, then the number of infected individuals moving from city i to city j is

$$\Delta I_{ij}^{in}(t) = \frac{I_i(t)m_{ij}(t)}{P_i}. \quad (7)$$

Also, the number of migrants leaving from city j is $\sum_{i=1}^{N} m_{ij}(t)$, and the number of infected cases that have migrated out of city j is

$$\Delta I_j^{out}(t) = \frac{I_j(t)\sum_{i=1}^{N} m_{ji}(t)}{P_j}, \quad (8)$$

where Pj(t) is the population of city j on day t. Thus, the increase in infected cases on day t in city j is given by

$$\Delta I_j(t) = \kappa_j(t)E_i(t) - \gamma(t)I_j(t) + \sum_{i=1}^{N} \Delta I_{ij}^{in}(t) - \Delta I_j^{out}(t)$$

$$= \kappa_j(t)E_i(t) - \gamma_j(t)I_j(t) + \sum_{i=1}^{N} \left(\frac{I_i(t)m_{ij}(t)}{P_i(t)} \right)$$

$$- \frac{I_j(t)\sum_{i=1}^{N} m_{ji}(t)}{P_j(t)} \tag{9}$$

where $\Delta Ij(t) = Ij(t+1) - Ij(t)$ and $kj(t)$ is the infection rate in city j on day t, i.e., the rate at which exposed individuals become infected. Moreover, infected individuals, once confirmed, would unlikely be able to migrate to another city. We thus implement this condition by writing (9) as

$$\Delta I_j(t) = \kappa_j(t)E_i(t) - \gamma_j(t)I_j(t)$$

$$+ k_I \left(\sum_{i=1}^{N} \left(\frac{I_i(t)m_{ij}(t)}{P_i(t)} \right) - \frac{I_j(t)\sum_{i=1}^{N} m_{ji}(t)}{P_j(t)} \right) \tag{10}$$

where $0 < kI << 1$ is a constant representing the possibility of an infected individual moving from one city to another. Likewise, incorporating the migrant dynamics, the increase in exposed individuals on day t in city j is

$$\Delta E_j(t) = \frac{\beta_j(t)}{N_j^s(t)}I_j(t)S_j(t) + \frac{\alpha_j(t)}{N_j^s(t)}E_j(t)S_j(t)$$

$$- \kappa_j(t)E_i(t) + \sum_{i=1}^{N} \left(\frac{E_i(t)m_{ij}(t)}{P_i(t)} \right)$$

$$- \frac{E_j(t)\sum_{i=1}^{N} m_{ji}(t)}{P_j(t)} \tag{11}$$

where $\Delta Ej(t) = Ej(t+1) - Ej(t)$, bj is the infection rate of susceptible individuals in city j, and aj is the infection rate of exposed individuals in city j. In a likewise fashion, we have

$$\Delta S_j(t) = -\frac{\beta_j(t)}{N_j^s(t)}I_j(t)S_j(t) - \frac{\alpha_j(t)}{N_j^s(t)}E_j(t)S_j(t)$$

$$+ \sum_{i=1}^{N} \left(\frac{S_i(t)m_{ij}(t)}{P_i(t)} \right) - \frac{S_j(t)\sum_{i=1}^{N} m_{ji}(t)}{P_j(t)} \tag{12}$$

where $\Delta Sj(t) = Sj(t+1) - Sj(t)$. Finally, we have

$$\Delta R_j(t) = \gamma_j(t)I_j(t), \tag{13}$$

where $\Delta Rj(t) = Rj(t+1) - Rj(t)$. In the above derivation, we should note that

the recovered individuals are assumed to stay in city j;

the recovery rates in different cities are assumed to be different due to varied quality of treatments and availability of medical facilities;

the recovery rates increase as time goes, as treatment methods are expected to improve gradually (i.e., taking gj(t) as a monotonically increasing function);

the eventual recovery rates in all cities will converge to the same constant $G \approx 1$.

In addition, due to intercity migration, the population of city j on day t would increase or decrease according to

$$\Delta P_j(t) = \sum_{i=1}^{N} \left(\frac{P_i(t)m_{ij}(t)}{P_i(t)} \right) - \frac{P_j(t) \sum_{i=1}^{N} m_{ji}(t)}{P_j(t)}$$

$$= \sum_{i=1}^{N} m_{ij}(t) - \sum_{i=1}^{N} m_{ji}(t)$$

(14)

where $\Delta P_j(t) = P_j(t+1) - P_j(t)$. Thus, the total susceptible population should be

$$\Delta N_j^s(t) = k_I \left(\sum_{i=1}^{N} \left(\frac{I_i(t)m_{ij}(t)}{P_i(t)} \right) - \frac{I_j(t) * \sum_{i=1}^{N} m_{ji}(t)}{P_j(t)} \right)$$

$$+ \sum_{i=1}^{N} \left(\frac{E_i(t)m_{ij}(t)}{P_i(t)} \right) - \frac{E_j(t) * \sum_{i=1}^{N} m_{ji}(t)}{P_j(t)}$$

$$+ \sum_{i=1}^{N} \left(\frac{S_i(t)m_{ij}(t)}{P_i(t)} \right) - \frac{S_j(t) \sum_{i=1}^{N} m_{ji}(t)}{P_j(t)}$$

(15)

where $\Delta N_j^S(t) = N_j^S(t+1) - N_j^S(t)$.

In summary, our modified SEIR model with consideration of human migration dynamics, for city *j*, is given by

$$\Delta I_j(t) = \kappa_j(t)E_i(t) - \gamma_j(t)I_j(t)$$

$$+ k_I \left(\sum_{i=1}^{N} \left(\frac{I_i(t)m_{ij}(t)}{P_i(t)} \right) - \frac{I_j(t) * \sum_{i=1}^{N} m_{ji}(t)}{P_j(t)} \right),$$

$$\Delta E_j(t) = \frac{\beta_j(t)}{N_j^s(t)}I_j(t)S_j(t) + \frac{\alpha_j(t)}{N_j^s(t)}E_j(t)S_j(t)$$

$$- \kappa_j(t)E_i(t) + \sum_{i=1}^{N} \left(\frac{E_i(t)m_{ij}(t)}{P_i(t)} \right)$$

$$- \frac{E_j(t)\sum_{i=1}^{N} m_{ji}(t)}{P_j(t)},$$

$$\Delta S_j(t) = -\frac{\beta_j(t)}{N_j^s(t)}I_j(t)S_j(t) - \frac{\alpha_j(t)}{N_j^s(t)}E_j(t)S_j(t)$$

$$+ \sum_{i=1}^{N} \left(\frac{S_i(t)m_{ij}(t)}{P_i(t)} \right) - \frac{S_j(t)\sum_{i=1}^{N} m_{ji}(t)}{P_j(t)}, \tag{16}$$

$$\Delta R_j(t) = \gamma_j(t)I_j(t),$$

$$\Delta P_j(t) = \sum_{i=1}^{N} m_{ij}(t) - \sum_{i=1}^{N} m_{ji}(t),$$

$$\Delta N_j^s(t) = k_I \left(\sum_{i=1}^{N} \left(\frac{I_i(t)m_{ij}(t)}{P_i(t)} \right) - \frac{I_j(t) * \sum_{i=1}^{N} m_{ji}(t)}{P_j(t)} \right)$$

$$+ \sum_{i=1}^{N} \left(\frac{E_i(t)m_{ij}(t)}{P_i(t)} \right) - \frac{E_j(t) * \sum_{i=1}^{N} m_{ji}(t)}{P_j(t)}$$

$$+ \sum_{i=1}^{N} \left(\frac{S_i(t)m_{ij}(t)}{P_i(t)} \right) - \frac{S_j(t)\sum_{i=1}^{N} m_{ji}(t)}{P_j(t)}$$

where subscript j denotes the city itself, and subscript i denotes another city from/to which people migrate on day t. Letting Xj(t) be the extended state vector, i.e., Xj(t) = [Sj(t) Ej(t) Ij(t) Rj(t) Pj(t) N_j^S(t)]T, we write the above difference equation as

$$\Delta X_j(t) = f(X_j, X_i, \mu_i) \tag{17}$$

where f(x) is the right side of (16), and μj is the set of parameters including aj, bj, gj, kj and dj. For computational convenience, we write (17) as

$$X_j(t+1) = X_j(t) + f(X_j, X_i, \mu_i) \tag{18}$$

In performing the data fitting, we assume aj, bj, gj, kj and dj are constants throughout the period of spreading, and the spreading begins at t0, at which N_j^S(t0) = dj Pj(t0).

Parameter Identification

The model represented by (18) describes the dynamics of the epidemic propagation with consideration of human migration dynamics. The parameters in model (18) are unknown and to be estimated from historical data. We solve this parameter identification problem via constrained nonlinear programming (CNLP), with the objective of finding an estimated growth trajectory that fits the data. An estimated number of infected cases of each city can be generated from (16) with unknown set qj, i.e.,

$$\theta_j = \{\alpha_j, \beta_j, \gamma_j, \kappa_j, \delta_j, I_{j,0}\} \qquad (19)$$

where Ij,0 = Ij(t0) is the initial number of infections in city j, and aj, bj, gj, kj and dj are parameters that determine the rates of spreading and recovery in city j. Then, the unknown set is Q = { q1, q2, ..., qK } essentially has 5K unknowns, where K is the number of cities, thus requiring an enormous effort of computation. Here, to gain computational efficiency, we assume that

all cities share one parameter set q = {a, b, k, g};

the numbers of initial infected and exposed individuals in city i are lIIi(t0) and lEIi(t0), respectively, where lI and lE are constant;

each city has an independent di.

Then, the size of the unknown set becomes computationally manageable, i.e.,

$$\Theta = \{\alpha, \beta, \kappa, \gamma, \delta_i, \lambda_I, \lambda_E\}.$$

Finally, the parameter estimation problem can be formulated as the following constrained nonlinear optimisation problem:

$$P_0: \min_{\Theta} \sum_{j=0}^{N} \left\| w_j (I(t_j) - \hat{I}(t_j)) \right\|_l$$

$$s.t. \begin{cases} \text{(i)} & \hat{x}(t+1) = \hat{x}(t) + F(\hat{x}(t)), \\ \text{(ii)} & \Theta_U \geq \Theta \geq \Theta_L, \end{cases} \qquad (20)$$

where F(.)represents model (18) and $\hat{x}(t) = [\ \hat{I}(t), \hat{R}(t), \hat{E}(t), \hat{S}(t), \hat{P}(t), \hat{N}^s(t)\ ]$ is the set of estimated variables, with unknown set Q, which is bounded between QL and QU. In this work, an inverse approach is taken to find the unknown parameters and states by solving (20). The Root Mean Square Percentage Error (RMSPE) is adopted as the criterion, i.e., fitting error, to measure the difference between the number of infected individuals generated by the model and the official daily infection data.

$$\text{RMSPE} = \sqrt{\frac{1}{K} \sum_{i=1} \sum_{j=1} \left(\frac{\hat{I}_i(t_j) - I_i(t_j)}{I_i(t_j)} \right)^2} \times 100\%,$$

(21)

where K is the number of cities to be evaluated.

Analysis and Results

We performed data fitting of the model, described by (18), using historical daily infection data provided by the National Health Commission of China, from January 24, 2020 to February 16, 2020. Prediction was performed on February 18, 2020 based on these early data. Our approach, as described in the previous section, was to apply constrained nonlinear programming to find the best set of estimates for the unknown parameters and states. Data fitting for all 367 cities were performed. Values were updated iteratively in the optimisation process. Moreover, since all parameters, like infection rates, were to be estimated by fitting data with the model, the integrity of the data became crucial. As the official Wuhan data were expected to deviate from the true values quite significantly during the early outbreak stage due to uncertainty in diagnosis and other issues related to reporting of the epidemic by the local government, we allowed the fitting errors for Wuhan to expand over a reasonable range, while the fitting errors for most other cities remained small. In addition, as the epidemic propagates in time, effective control measures and improved public education would reduce the infection rates for the susceptible and exposed individuals, making these parameters time varying in reality. Nonetheless, our fitting has assumed these parameters being constant during the short fitting period for computational simplicity.

The propagation profiles, in terms of the number of infected individuals and estimated number of exposed individuals, for all 367 cities were estimated. Shown in Figure 4.4 are the results for 15 selected cities. This model could also provide projections of the number of infected and exposed individuals in the next 200 days, as shown in Figure 4.5, which clearly showed that the daily infection would reach a peak sooner or later. By running the identification algorithm, we identified the optimal parameter set as a = 0.5869, b = 0.8949, k = 0.1008, and g = 0.0602. From the estimated propagation profiles of the COVID-19 epidemic for all 367 cities, we have the following findings:

- For most cities, the infection numbers would peak between mid-February to early March 2020, as shown in Figure 4.6(a).

- The peak number of infected individuals would be between 1,000 to 5,000 for cities in Hubei, and that outside Hubei would be below 500, as shown in Figure 4.6(b).

- At the end, about 0.8%, less than 0.1% and less than 0.01% of the population would get infected in Wuhan, Hubei Province and the rest of China, respectively, as presented in Figure 4.6(c). Translating to actual figures, for most cities outside and within Hubei Province (except Wuhan), the total number of infected individuals was expected to be fewer than 300 and 4000, respectively, as shown in Figure 4.6(d).

Figure 4.4. Official number of infected individuals and estimated number of infected individuals in 15 selected cities in China (upper), and estimated number of exposed individuals (lower)

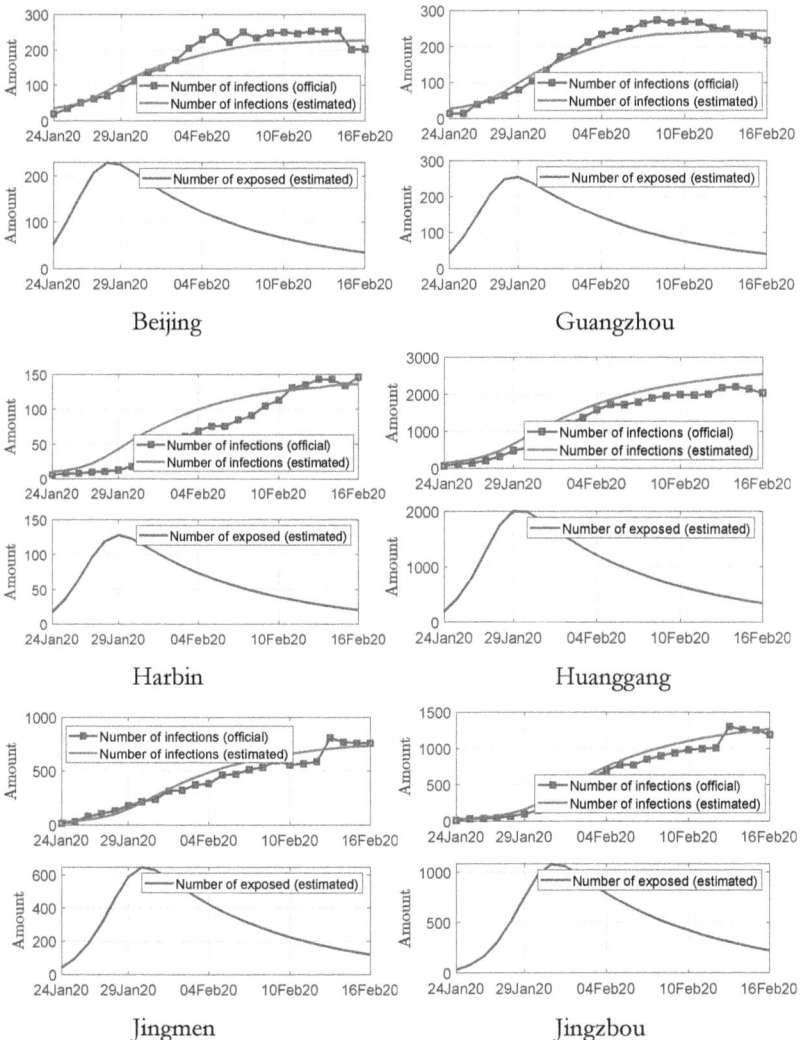

Beijing

Guangzhou

Harbin

Huanggang

Jingmen

Jingzhou

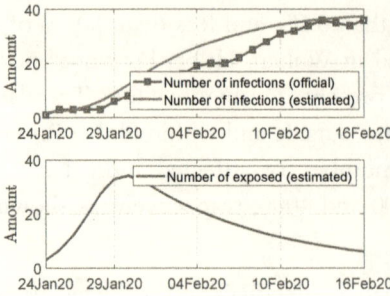
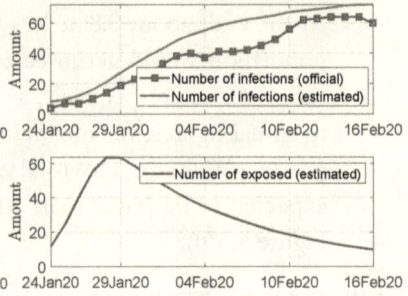

Lianyungang   Nanjing

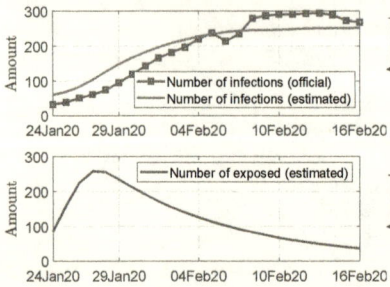
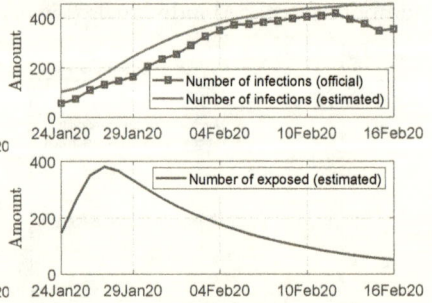

Shanghai   Shenzhen

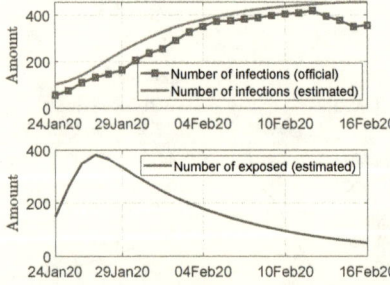
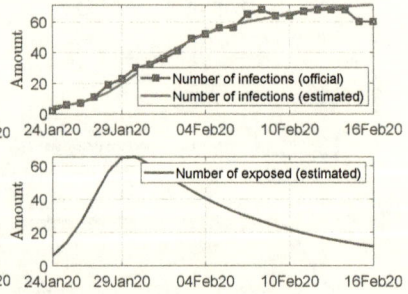

Chongqing   Suzhou

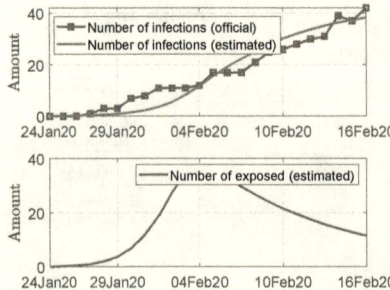
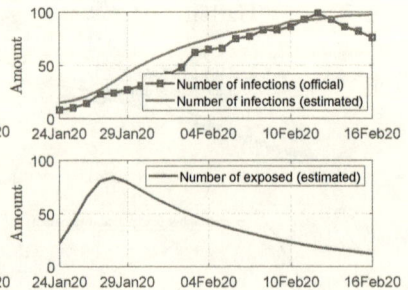

Tangshan   Tianjin

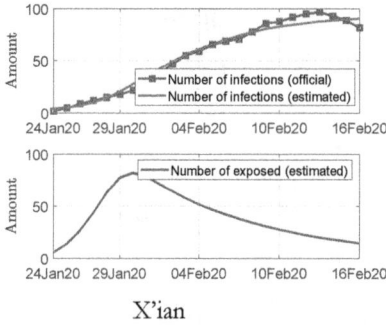

X'ian

Figure 4.5. Prediction of the number of infected (upper) and exposed individuals (lower) in 15 selected cities in China in the next 150 days from February 16, 2020.

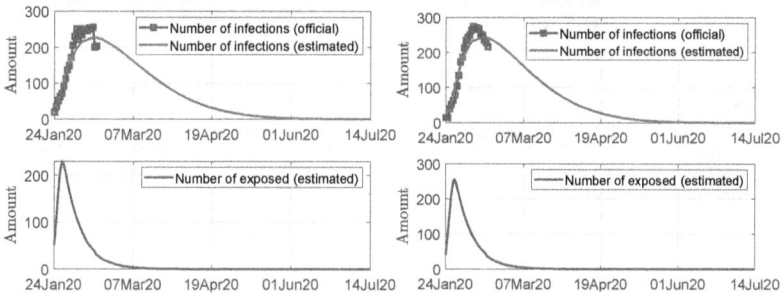

Beijing   Guangzhou

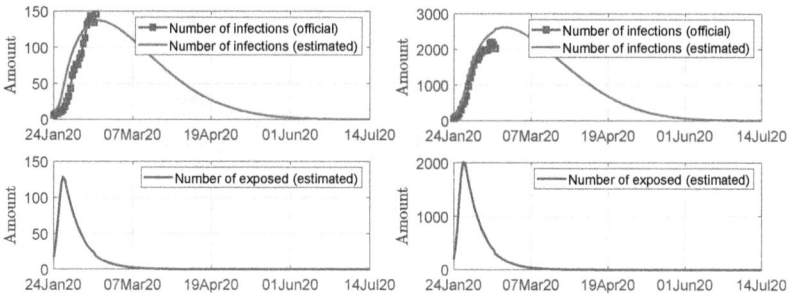

Harbin   Huanggang

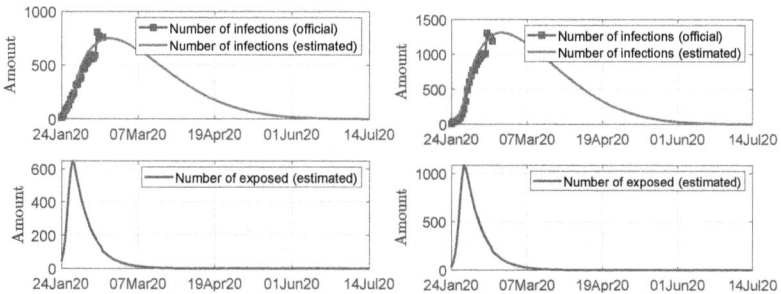

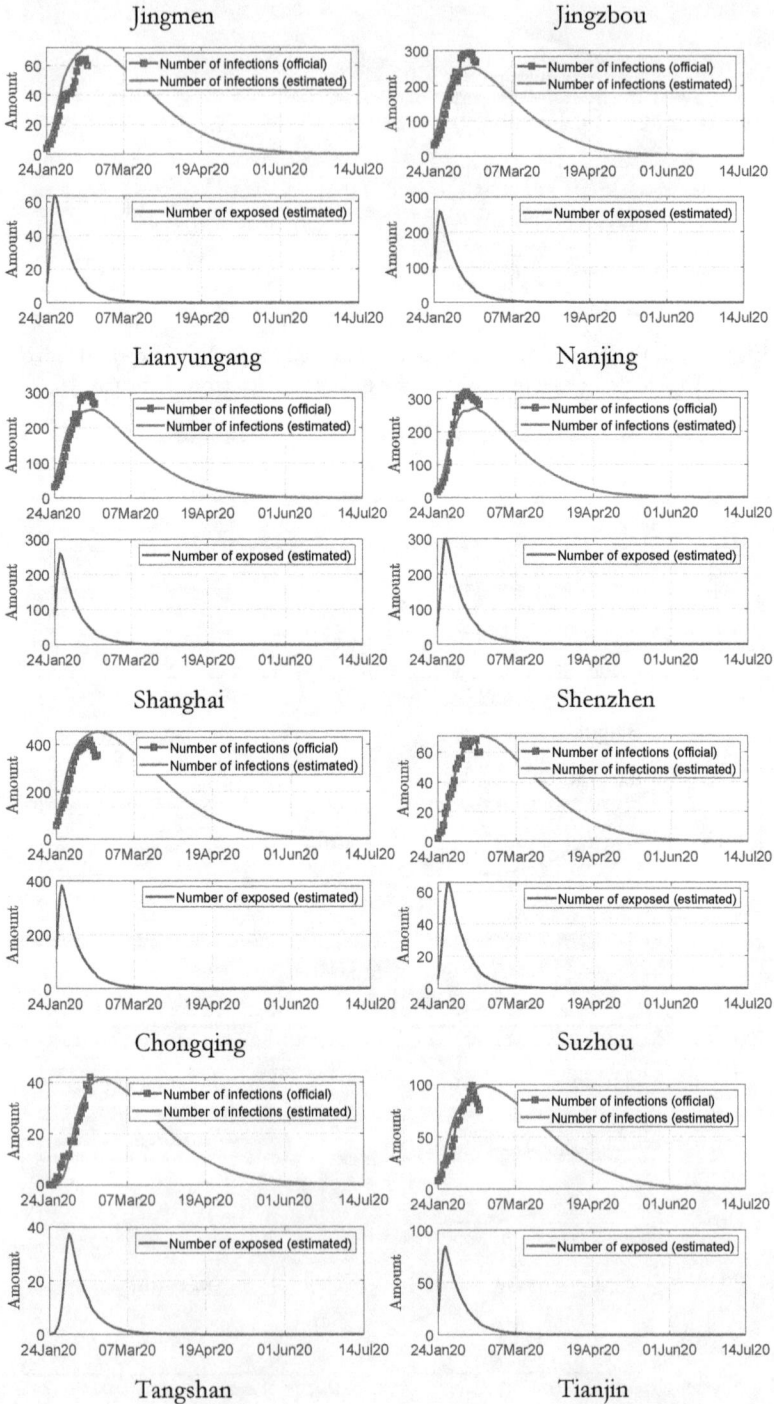

Jingmen

Jingzhou

Lianyungang

Nanjing

Shanghai

Shenzhen

Chongqing

Suzhou

Tangshan

Tianjin

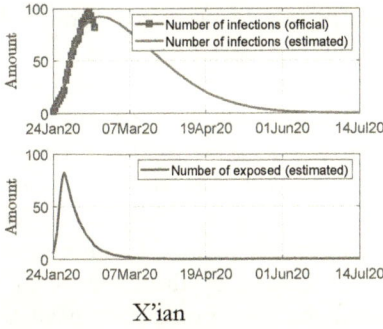

X'ian

Figure 4.6. (a) Distribution of (a) peak time; (b) peak number of infections; (c) proportion of the population eventually infected in a city; (d) total number of individuals eventually infected in a city.

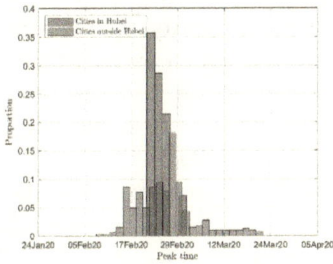

(a)

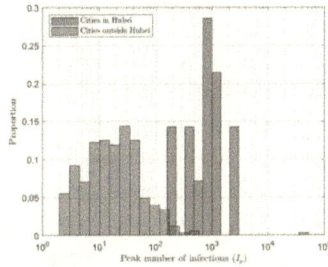

(b)

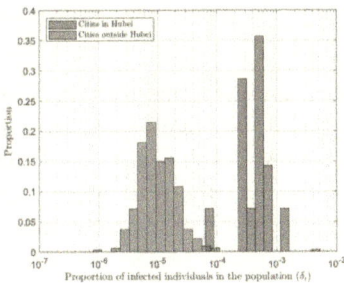

(c)

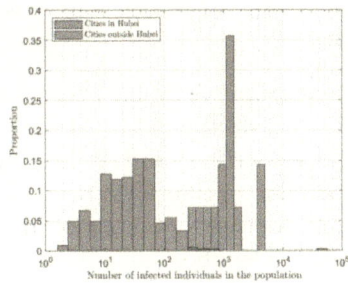

(d)

Interpretations

Opinions diverged on the estimated extent of the outbreak of the new coronavirus disease (COVID-19). While there were pure speculations, there were also predictions based on rigorous study of the spreading dynamics. Different models used for prediction and different assumptions made regarding the transmission process would lead to different results and quite diverged conclusions. For instance, in February 2020, an AI-powered

43

simulation run had predicted 2.5 billion people to be infected in 45 days (Koetsier, 2020). Academics in Hong Kong expected 1.4 million eventually infected in the city of 7.5 million people. Our results, however, did not seem to agree with such predictions. In fact, our results were expected to be optimistic, under normal circumstances, in the sense that the projected severity and duration of the epidemic were valid provided stringent measures continued to be in place to curb the spread of the virus, especially before mid-March. On the positive side, active intervention would continue to be implemented and a level of vigilance maintained by the majority of the population. Actual data have also shown that our predictions have been highly consistent with reality. Infection peaks in various cities in China did not occur later than the predicted times.

Furthermore, the effectiveness of medical treatment has kept being improved and the recovery rate has increased since March 2020. Thus, as our simulation was based on data collected until mid-February, the recovery rate could be under-estimated. Should the recovery rate increase by 0.0005 each day, namely, the number of daily recovered individuals increases by 1% of the total number of infected individuals every 20 days, most cities in China would have zero infection case by the end of June 2020. However, as the world is connected and unless strict travel bans were in place (currently most countries still allow their own citizens to return), possibility exists for infected individuals including those who are asymptomatic to move from city to city, however small in quantity. Second and third waves of outbreaks could not be ruled out! A high level of vigilance should be maintained to prevent the continuous spread of the virus, especially via the active transportation network.

Furthermore, we should stress that this work was completed on February 19, 2020 (medRxiv 10.1101/2020.02.18.20024570), and we used a short historical epidemic spread and migration data to develop the model and the corresponding system identification algorithm. At the time of performing this work, there was no attempt in combining SEIR model, migration data and system identification techniques to analyse and predict the spread of COVID-19. The results thus have important indicative values on the effectiveness of using limited initial outbreak data in predicting pandemic progression.

Conclusion

The Novel Coronavirus Disease 2019 (COVID-19) epidemic has initially hit China hard. While the virus began to spread to other countries from February 2020, the extent of the outbreak in China remained to be severe in comparison to other countries for much of March and April 2020. Prediction of the severity and duration of the epidemic provided essential information for illuminating social and non-pharmaceutical interventions. However, prediction with the needed level of accuracy was a non-trivial task. In this work, we employed human migration data to provide information on intercity travel that was crucial to the transmission of the novel coronavirus disease from its epicentre Wuhan to other parts of China.

The model described in this chapter was essentially the classic SEIR model, with intercity travel data supplying the essential information about the number of infected, exposed and recovered individuals moving between different cities. All parameters of the model, including infection rates, recovery rates, and eventual percentage of infected population for 367 cities in China, were identified by fitting the official data collected up to mid-February with the model using a constrained nonlinear programming procedure. Using these parameters, predictions of the number of exposed individuals in 367 cities as well as projections into the next 200 days were made. Our model, however, did not consider the contact network topology that would be necessary if details of the transmission process, such as superspreading events, were to be captured. Nonetheless, our model provided a highly consistent estimation of the propagation of average numbers of exposed, infected and recovered individuals, despite missing details of fluctuation (e.g., sudden surge due to a superspreading event).

The main conclusion of our study is that provided stringent control measures including travel restriction continued to be in place, the COVID-19 epidemic spreading was expected to peak between mid-February to early March 2020, with about 0.8%, less than 0.1% and less than 0.01% of the population eventually infected in Wuhan, Hubei Province and the rest of China, respectively. As the effectiveness of treatment continued to improve and in the absence of imported cases, our model predicted that the COVID-19 epidemic in China would end by June 2020. However, possibilities of a second wave of outbreaks may exist as intercity travel is still permitted, e.g., homebound travel from regions which are still at different stages of the pandemic progression. It is thus advisable to maintain a high level of vigilance by the public as well as a high level of preparedness for reactivating stringent control measures by government authorities.

Acknowledgement

CZ was supported by National Science Foundation of China Project 61703355 and Science and Technology Program of Guangzhou, China 201904010224. CKT was supported City University of Hong Kong under Special Fund 9380114.

References

Baidu Migration. (2020). URL https://http://qianxi.baidu.com/.

Boguná M, Pastor-Satorras R, & Vespignani A. (2003). Absence of epidemic threshold in scale-free networks with degree correlations. Phys Rev Lett 90(2): 028701.

Chakrabarti D, Wang Y, Wang C, Leskovec J, & Faloutsos C. (2008). Epidemic thresholds in real networks. ACM Trans Inform Syst Security 10(4): 1.

Colizza V, Barrat A, Barthélemy M, & Vespignani A. (2006). The role of the airline transportation network in the prediction and predictability of global epidemics. Proc. National Acad Sci of the United States of America 103(7): 2015–2020.

Diekmann O, Heesterbeek H, & Britton T. (2013). Mathematical Tools for Understanding Infectious Disease Dynamics. Princeton University Press.

Gross T, D'Lima CJ, & Blasius B. (2006). Epidemic dynamics on an adaptive network. Phys Rev Lett 96(20): 208701.

Li A, Guan X, Wu P, Wang X, Zhou L, Tong Y, et al. (2020). Early transmission dynamics in Wuhan China of novel coronavirus-infected pneumonia, New Eng J Med DOI: 10.1056/NEJMoa2001316.

Pastor-Satorras R & Vespignani A. (2001). Epidemic spreading in scale-free networks. Phys Rev Lett 86(14): 3200.

Small M & Tse CK. (2005). Small world and scale free network model of transmission of SARS. Int J Bifurc Chaos 15(5): 1745–1756.

Small M, Tse CK, & Walker D. (2006). Super-spreaders and the rate of transmission of the SARS virus. Physica D 215: 146–158.

Wang Y, Chakrabarti D, Wang C, & Faloutsos C. (2003). Epidemic spreading in real networks: An eigenvalue viewpoint. Proc IEEE Int Symp Reliable Distributed Syst. 25–34.

Du Z, Wang L, Cauchemez S, Xu X, Wang X, Cowling BJ, & Meyers LA. (2020). Risk of transportation of 2019 novel coronavirus disease from Wuhan to other cities in China. Emerging Infectious Disease 26(5) DOI: 10.3201/eid2601.200146.

Koetsier J. (2020). AI predicts coronavirus could infect 2.5 billion and kill 53 million. URL https://www.healthexec.com/topics/care-delivery/ai-predicts-25b-coronavirus-infections.

CHAPTER 5

THE STUDY OF THE EFFECTS OF MOBILITY TRENDS ON THE STATISTICAL MODELS OF THE COVID-19 VIRUS SPREADING

David Gondauri and Mikheil Batiashvili

Introduction

The history of the Pandemics makes a significant impact on the memory and behavior of the affected communities. The outbreak of the COVID-19 virus in Wuhan, Hubei Province, China was followed by the rapid spreading from its origin (Peeters Grietens, 2015). For the time being the causative virus has been named as a severe acute respiratory syndrome coronavirus 2 (SARS-CoV-2) and the relevant infected disease has been named as coronavirus disease 2019 (COVID-19) by the World Health Organization respectively. Conferring to the daily report of the World Health Organization, the epidemic of SARS-CoV-2 had registered 118,319 cases and 4,292 deaths in 113 countries according to the reported numbers by March 11, 2020 and the World Health Organization declared the outbreak of a pandemic (Gondauri et al., 2020). Following the outbreak significant behavioral, clinical, and state interventions have been undertaken to ease the epidemic and prevent the transmittal of the virus in remaining human populations in China and worldwide. It remains unclear how these governmental interventions, including travel restrictions, affected COVID-19 spread in China. We use real-time mobility data from Wuhan and detailed case data including travel history to elucidate the role of case introduction on transmission in cities across China and determine the impact of the imposed control measures. The spatial distribution of COVID-19 cases in China was explained well by human mobility data. Following the execution of the government control measures, this correlation of the spreading dropped and growth rates became negative in most places, although shifts in the demographics of the reported cases were still indicative of local chains of transmission outside Wuhan. The following study shows that the radical and sever control procedures employed in China substantially mitigated the spread of COVID-19 virus (Kraamer et al., 2020). Limiting the social contacts of these individuals was crucial for COVID-19 control, because patients with no or mild symptoms can spread the virus (Peeters Grietens, 2015).

As it is known from the previous examples, the importance of human mobility for malaria elimination was evident in earlier elimination attempts. However, malaria re-emerged due to the failed surveillance systems that had to account the movements of the affected human populations (Peeters Grietens, 2015).

Human mobility is a major factor in the spread of vector-borne diseases such as dengue even on the short scale corresponding to intra-city distances. In this study, we finally discuss the advantages and the limits of mobile phone data and potential alternatives for assessing valuable mobility patterns for modeling vector-borne diseases outbreaks in the cities (Massaro et al., 2019). However, it is important consumers perceive the risks of a pandemic strongly, they can influence the beliefs of those around them about the risks they are facing, and it also promotes their attitude to cope with threats from the external environment (Long and Khoi, 2020).

Thus, it is important to study the connection between human mobility and the spread of viral infection. Specifically, we aimed to investigate whether there was a correlation between Mobility Trends and the spread of Covid-19 virus.

Materials and Methods

For this purpose, we used the Mobility Trends from the reports of the company Apple. The given reports are published daily and reflect requests for directions in Apple Maps. Privacy is one of our basic values, so the maps doesn't associate the user's data with the individual Apple ID, and Apple doesn't keep a history of where the user has been traveling. In many countries/regions and cities, relative traffic volume has increased since January 13th, consistent with the normal, seasonal usage of Apple Maps application. Day of week effects are important to normalize as the individual uses this data. Data that is sent from users' devices to the maps service is associated with random, rotating identifiers so Apple doesn't have a profile of individuals movements and its search history. Apple Maps has no demographic information about the application users, so any statements about the representativeness of the usage against the overall population cannot be made.

Data on confirmed cases of the Covid-19 virus transmission have been obtained from the World Health Organization's official daily reports. The data covers the number of people infected with COVID-19 virus since January 22 to April 14, 2020. As of January 22, there were 580 cases of reported infections, and as of April 14, the number reached 1,844,863, Including 71,779 Total confirmed cases.

We calculated the results, and analyzed the data using regression slope and Pearson correlation. The regression slope method implies how much of a second variable changes by 1% of one variable. We have observed the global impact of pedestrian, machine and transit traffic on the impact of the spread of the virus, in particular the 1% change in the cumulative number of confirmed infected cases. Correlation coefficients are scaled such that they range from −1 to +1, where 0 indicates that there is no linear or monotonic association, and the relationship gets stronger and ultimately approaches a straight line (Pearson correlation) (Schober et al., 2018).

Pearson's product moment correlation coefficient is denoted as ϱ for a population parameter and as r for a sample statistic. It is used when both variables being studied are normally distributed. This coefficient is affected by extreme values, which may exaggerate or dampen the strength of relationship, and is therefore inappropriate when either or both variables are not normally distributed. For a correlation between variables x and y, the formula for calculating the sample Pearson's correlation coefficient is given by

$$r = \frac{\sum_{i=1}^{n} (x_i - x)(y_i - y)}{\sqrt{\left[\sum_{i=1}^{n} (x_i - \bar{x})^2\right]\left[\sum_{i=1}^{n} (y_i - \bar{y})^2\right]}}$$

where xi and yi are the values of x and y for the ith individual (Mukaka, 2012). We even used the Pearson correlation to determine the correlation between Mobility Trends and the total amount of infection.

For the study purposed, we have also selected the 8 countries which as of date April 15, 2020, have the highest numbers of the confirmed cases of the Corona Virus. Those countries are: USA (Total confirmed cases – 578,268), Spain (Total confirmed cases – 172,541), Italy (Total confirmed cases – 162,488), Germany (Total confirmed cases – 12,758), France (Total confirmed cases – 102,533), The United Kingdom (Total confirmed cases – 93,877), Turkey (Total confirmed cases – 65,111) and Belgium (Total confirmed cases – 31,119). At the same time, the Mobility Trends of these countries were recorded by the Apple. We also selected one additional country - New Zealand, which was characterized by a reliable decrease in the spread of the virus (Total cases – 1,386; Daily cases - 20; Total recovered cases - 728). The data covers the number of Mobility Trends from January 13 to April 14, 2020. The data were divided into two periods before the pandemic (before March 11, 2020) and after the pandemic. We calculated the slope, correlation, and determination coefficients between intensity of walking, driving, transit and the prevalence of the virus according to the data of the given countries from January 22 to March 11 and from March 11 to April 14.

Limitation of the study provided we considered only a linear relationship between the variables. Naturally there are other factors that influence the number of infected cases that we disregarded in the study.

Results and Findings

The study is based on the COVID-19 statistical study based on Apple Maps data, which shows the movement of citizens by walking, by driving and transit as globally as in the following countries: USA, Italy, Spain, France, Germany, The United Kingdom, Belgium, Turkey, New Zealand.

Figure 5.1. The cumulative number of globally confirmed cases of globally infected Covid-19 virus is given by day from January 22 to April 14; Graphically, the change in the number of pedestrians (Yellow columns), cars (Green columns), transit traffic (Red columns).

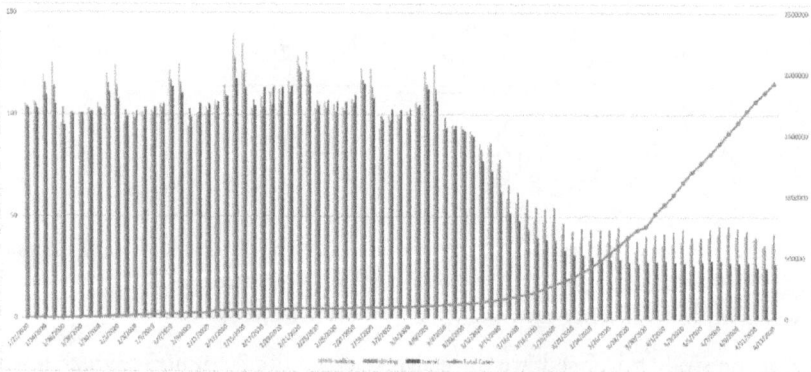

Walking - the volume of the spread of the virus. According to the statistical model, between January 22 and March 11, before the announcement of the pandemic, the slope between the number of pedestrians and the spread of the virus was 2.56%, which means that when the spread of the virus increased by 1%, the intensity of pedestrians increased. By 2.56%. As for March 12-April 14, Slope is already negative among the already mentioned variables - 2.61 times. The results already indicate that in the second phase of the virus spread (March 12 - April 14) in parallel with the 1% increase in the spread of the virus, the intensity of pedestrians decreased by 2.61 times. As for the correlation between the presented variables, it was -75% for the mentioned period, and its determination coefficient (R ^ 2) is 56.28.

Driving- the volume of the spread of the virus. From January 22 until the announcement of the pandemic (March 11), the slope between the intensity of traffic and the extent of the spread of the virus was -1,156 times. This indicates that during this period, when the spread of the virus increased by 1%, the intensity of traffic increased by 1,156 times. As for March 12-April 14, Slope is already negative among the already mentioned variables - 2.61 times. In the second phase of the spread of the virus (March 12 - April 14) in parallel with the 1% increase in the spread of the virus, the intensity of traffic decreased by 3.18 times. As for the correlation between the presented variables for the mentioned period, it was -77.9%, and its determination coefficient ($R \wedge 2$) is 60.69%.

Transit - the volume of the spread of the virus. During the study it was identified that between the January 22 and March 11 (March 11), the intensity of transit traffic and the prevalence of the virus, the number of slips was 2.76. This data indicates that during this period, when the prevalence of the virus increased by 1%, the intensity of transit traffic increased 2.76 times during the given period. As for the March 12 - April 14, the slot is already negative - 2.45 times. In the second phase of the spread of the virus (March 12 - April 14), along with the 1% increase in the spread of the virus, the intensity of transit traffic decreased by 2.45 times. As for the correlation between the presented variables for the mentioned period, it was -78.2%, with its determination coefficient ($R \wedge 2$) is 61.12%.

The table below shows the slope, correlation, and determination coefficients between pedestrians, traffic, transit intensity, and the prevalence of the virus by countries from January 22 to March 22 (March 11) and March 12 to April 14.

Table 5.1 shows that the slope and correlation coefficients are both positive and negative. From 22.01.2020 to 14.04.2020, the maximum value of the positive slope coefficient between the US pedestrian traffic (1.04 times) and the intensity of traffic (2,653 times) and the prevalence of the virus. And Spain has the highest positive ratio between the intensity of transit traffic and the spread of the virus in Spain (2,985 times). 22.01.2020 - 14.04.2020 The maximum value of the negative slope coefficient is between Turkey in terms of pedestrian traffic (-6,312 times), Italy - in terms of traffic intensity (-8,074 times) and the prevalence of the virus. And the highest negative ratio between the transit traffic intensity and the prevalence of the virus in Belgium (-9.560 times).

Table 5.1 shows that the slope and correlation coefficients are both positive and negative. From 22.01.2020 to 14.04.2020, the maximum value of the positive slope coefficient between the US pedestrian traffic (1.04 times) and the intensity of traffic (2,653 times) and the prevalence of the virus. And Spain has the highest positive ratio between the intensity of transit traffic and the spread of the virus in Spain (2,985 times). 22.01.2020 - 14.04.2020 The maximum value of the negative slope coefficient is between Turkey in terms of pedestrian traffic (-6,312 times), Italy - in terms of traffic intensity (-8,074 times) and the prevalence of the virus. And the highest negative ratio between the transit traffic intensity and the prevalence of the virus in Belgium (-9.560 times).

Table 5.1. Slope, correlation and determination coefficients obtained by Apple Maps traffic intensity by the country.

country	Date	slope Total Cases to			Correl Total Cases to			R^2		
		walking	driving	transit	walking	driving	transit	walking	driving	transit
USA	22.01.2020-11.03.2020	1.040	2.653	-1.415	-0.608	-0.654	-0.682	0.370	0.427	0.465
	12.03.2020-14.04.2020	-6.099	-6.449	-5.096						
Spain	22.01.2020-11.03.2020	-2.097	-5.102	2.985	-0.706	-0.737	-0.723	0.499	0.543	0.523
	12.03.2020-14.04.2020	-1.564	-2.140	-1.951						
Italy	22.01.2020-11.03.2020	-6.174	-8.074	-6.297	-0.720	-0.768	-0.753	0.518	0.589	0.567
	12.03.2020-14.04.2020	-0.783	-0.210	-4.735						
France	22.01.2020-11.03.2020	-2.665	-5.698	0.353	-0.729	-0.759	-0.765	0.532	0.576	0.585
	12.03.2020-14.04.2020	-1.581	-1.692	-1.387						
Germany	22.01.2020-11.03.2020	-1.887	-7.095	1.243	-0.597	-0.733	-0.734	0.356	0.537	0.538
	12.03.2020-14.04.2020	-1.498	-3.835	-3.109						
UK	22.01.2020-11.03.2020	-0.780	-1.823	-7.831	-0.638	-0.751	-0.725	0.407	0.564	0.525
	12.03.2020-14.04.2020	-3.561	-3.487	-2.391						
Belgium	22.01.2020-11.03.2020	-2.623	-4.972	-9.560	-0.538	-0.676	-0.693	0.290	0.457	0.480
	12.03.2020-14.04.2020	-0.532	-2.966	-2.499						
New Zealand	28.02.2020 - 14.04.2020	-3.676	-2.635	-2.421	-0.831	-0.868	-0.840	0.690	0.753	0.705
Turkey	28.02.2020 - 14.04.2020	-6.312	-6.547	0.000	-0.617	-0.680	0.000	0.380	0.462	0.000

During this period, the correlation coefficient in all presented directions is negative. New Zealand has the highest negative correlation between pedestrians (-83.07%), vehicle traffic intensity (86.8%) and the prevalence of the virus. Therefore, their determination coefficient (R^2) was 69.01% and 75.34%, respectively.

Conclusion

Social distancing and lock down will benefit the local and international community. Moreover, it has been suggested that evacuations may contribute to the international spread of a highly contagious disease of pandemic potential (Musinguzi and Asamoah, 2020). Also to be considered, significant disparities in social determinants of health exist between the rural and urban areas. They are likely to increase mortality rate to COVID-19 if the disease reaches the rural areas. Deliberate and proactive measures are needed acutely to prevent the spread of this disease to rural areas. Contingency plans must be in place to deal with the disease should it eventually get there (Ameh et al., 2020). "Contamination due to contact with the infected person" is the main responsible factor behind the pandemic COVID-19. Also, in this investigation we get an optimal model by which we can monitor the death from Coronavirus within the affected person continuously. By Doctors opinion, Literature review and Media Survey was selected three risk factors of Coronavirus namely Verbal contamination, contamination through eatables, and contamination due to contact with the infected person (Majumder et al., 2020). The study showed that elderly patients and those with comorbidities are most susceptible for this infection, and will have the worst prognosis (Dakhil and Farhan, 2020).

Thus in this study, in the conclusion it should be noted that the intensity of pedestrians, traffic and transit traffic during the study period, on average, after 15-20 days, affected the spread of the virus. If there was a positive slope and correlation coefficient between the variables presented in the period 22.01.2020 - 11.03.2020 (before the announcement of the pandemic), in the period 12.03.2020 - 14.04.2020 (after the announcement of the pandemic) the slope and correlation coefficients received negative values between the study variables, which indicates That on average, after 15-20 days, Due to the intensity of the movement, the center of the virus spreading is identified, and the intensity of the movement itself is decreased.

For future research, these correlation studies will play an important role in further influencing mobility trends in the prevention of various infectious diseases, as well as socio-economic impact, health, and ecosystem sustainability in the post-epidemic period.

References

Ameh, G. et al. (2020). Rural America and Coronavirus Epidemic: Challenges and Solutions. European Journal of Environment and Public Health, 4(2), em0040. https://doi.org/10.29333/ejeph/8200

Chen S., Yang J., Yang W., Wang C., Bärnighausen T. (2020). COVID-19 control in China during mass population movements at New Year. Lancet. 2020; 395, 764–766. doi:10.1016/S0140-6736(20)30421-9

Dakhil ZA, Farhan HA. (2020). Cardiovascular Impacts of COVID-19 Pandemic: From Presentation to Management: Current and Future Perspectives. J Clin Exp Invest. 2020;11(3):em00739. https://doi.org/10.5799/jcei/7941.

Gondauri D., Mikautadze E., Batiashvili M. (2020). Research on COVID-19 Virus Spreading Statistics based on the Examples of the Cases from Different Countries. Electron J Gen Med. 2020;17(4):em209. https://doi.org/10.29333/ejgm/7869

Kraemer M.U.G. et al. (2020). The effect of human mobility and control measures on the COVID-19 epidemic in China. *Science*. 2020; 25 Mar: eabb4218. DOI:

10.1126/science.abb4218

Long NN, Khoi BH. (2020). An Empirical Study about the Intention to Hoard Food during COVID-19 Pandemic. EURASIA J MATH SCI T. 2020;16(7), em1857. https://doi.org/10.29333/ejmste/8207

Majumder P, Biswas P, Majumder S. (2020). Application of New TOPSIS Approach to Identify the Most Significant Risk Factor and Continuous Monitoring of Death of COVID-19. Electron J Gen Med. 2020;17(6): em234. https://doi.org/10.29333/ejgm/7904

Massaro E., Kondor D. & Ratti C. (2019). Assessing the interplay between human mobility and mosquito borne diseases in urban environments. Sci Rep. 2019; 9, 16911. https://doi.org/10.1038/s41598-019-53127-z

Mukaka MM. (2012). Statistics corner: A guide to appropriate use of correlation coefficient in medical research. *Malawi Med J.* 2012; 24(3):69–71. PMID: 23638278

Musinguzi G., Asamoah BO. (2020). The Science of Social Distancing and Total Lock Down: Does it Work? Whom does it Benefit?. Electron J Gen Med. 2020; 17(6):em230. https://doi.org/10.29333/ejgm/7895

Peeters Grietens K. et al. (2015). Characterizing Types of Human Mobility to Inform Differential and Targeted Malaria Elimination Strategies in Northeast Cambodia. *Sci Rep.* 2015; 5, 16837. https://doi.org/10.1038/srep16837

Schober P., Boer Ch., Schwarte L.A. (2018). Correlation Coefficients: Appropriate Use and Interpretation. Anesthesia & Analgesia. 2018; 126(5):1763-1768 doi:10.1213/ANE.0000000000002864

CHAPTER 6

HUMAN MOBILITY, COVID-19 AND POLICY RESPONSES: THE RIGHTS AND CLAIMS-MAKING OF MIGRANT DOMESTIC WORKERS

Smriti Rao, Sarah Gammage, Julia Arnold and Elizabeth J. Anderson

Introduction

It is clear that the novel coronavirus (COVID-19) attacks our biological and socio-economic vulnerabilities. Sharp variations in mortality rates have forced us to acknowledge pre-existing inequalities of class, race and gender in the ability to 'be safe, be well' even as a disproportionate amount of the economic pain and suffering of this crisis is being visited upon the poorest and most vulnerable. One unique feature of the COVID-19 response is the need to curb mobility to reduce disease transmission. These curbs on human mobility (notably not matched by curbs on flows of capital) directly impact the vast flows of human migration that the global economy is built upon today. And while the bulk of public attention and policy intervention in most countries has been focused on domestic effects, international migrant workers have long been 'essential but disposable' workers of the kind most affected by the health and economic effects of the pandemic.

In the aftermath of COVID-19, while on the one hand many migrants lost their livelihoods, the ability to draw on migrant workers to continue to provide essential goods and services emerged as an important strategy that countries used to manage these lockdowns. The 'essential and disposable' nature of migrant workers, including MDWs, allowed some countries to implement less stringent lockdowns by exposing migrant workers, rather than citizens, to the greater risks of working through the lockdowns. In fact, migrant communities in the Gulf and in the Americas have seen a large number of COVID-19 cases compared to the general populations in the same countries (Appendix).

Migrant domestic workers in particular constitute a core of workers most at risk of suffering negative health and economic impacts, and least likely to be assisted by domestic policy responses during the pandemic (Varia, 2006, ILO, 2016a; WHO, 2017; Pérez Orozco, 2016). They are a uniquely intersectional category of workers who labor in a sector that frequently extends beyond the realm of labor law and social protection. Gendered notions of who can perform this labor mean that almost 75% of domestic workers across the world are women, and often women of color, so that the vulnerabilities and exclusions they experience are gendered, classed, and raced (ILO, 2016a, Oliviera, 2017). Unlike migrant domestic workers who are citizens, the rights of MDWs are further circumscribed by immigration law and practice (Kontos, 2013). And in comparison to migrant workers more generally, migrant domestic workers are much more likely to be isolated as workers, working alone for, and in some cases living with, private employers.

Understanding how and when MDWs have attempted to seek protections from host and home countries in this time of heightened isolation and vulnerability provides insight into rights and claims-making in the gray areas of global governance during crises (Boris and Unden, 2017). Where migrant domestic workers become essential extensions of care systems with different degrees of enfranchisement and inclusion or recognition, it is important to make their work visible and support this claims-making (Altman and Pannell, 2012).

We explore these issues through a textual analysis of interviews we conducted with 15 Subject Matter Experts (SMEs) engaged with and representing migrant women workers in the labor movement and in health and humanitarian organizations in key migration corridors. We interviewed SMEs in, or associated with, a number of host countries (Hong Kong, Lebanon, Qatar, Jordan, Kuwait, United States, Spain, Italy, Germany, Costa Rica and Canada), as well as some associated sending countries (Philippines, Bangladesh, Nepal, Morocco, Mexico). The host countries were chosen to be representative of major migration corridors for domestic migrant workers who are concentrated in North America, Western Southern and Northern Europe, and the Gulf States (ILO, 2016a). We recruited SMEs voluntarily through networks such as the Women in Migration Network, the Solidarity Center, Mercy Corps, Human Rights Watch, the International Domestic Workers Federation, the International Labor Organization and the International Organization for Migration.

Our analysis here is updated as of the last week of May 2020. At this stage, COVID-19 had spread the most in relatively high-income countries, influencing our choice of case study countries. In most countries, COVID-19 lockdowns/mobility restrictions had not yet been eased by the last week of May, so our analysis covers a phase of particularly pervasive lockdowns.

Our qualitative interviews confirm the essential-but-disposable nature of MDWs. We show that outcomes for migrant domestic workers have tended to be better where the pre-COVID-19 infrastructure of social provisioning was stronger. The relationship to the larger environment of democracy is complex. While more authoritarian regimes in host countries are also more likely to restrict the rights and mobility of MDWs, this is not necessarily the case, and opportunities may have opened up for more coordinated claims-making in home and host countries as a result of the pandemic.

Migrant workers, social distancing and social provisioning: Understanding the impacts of COVID-19

From 1980 to 2019, the number of global migrants more than doubled from 101 million to 272 million (IOM, 2020). Currently, women make up almost half of all international migrants, accounting for almost 80% of migrants from some countries (Donato and Gabaccia, 2015, ILO, 2016). Of the 150 million migrant workers worldwide, around 8% are domestic workers in private homes, a figure that rises to 13% for women migrant workers. Almost one in five domestic workers across the world are migrants, with that share rising to 83% of all domestic workers in Arab states, 71% in North America and 55% in Western, Southern and Northern Europe (ILO, 2016).

The essential nature of the work MDWs undertake begins with its importance in sustaining patterns of high labor force participation for women and men in high-income countries, as they outsource cleaning, cooking and direct care of elderly and children to MDWs. Demographic changes in high-income countries have contributed to an increase in demand for MDWs over the least two decades. Aging populations increase the need for elder care, and relatively high women's work force participation rates, together with relatively inflexible gender divisions of labor, increase demand for paid care labor. These trends are unlikely to be reversed in the aftermath of the COVID-19 crisis. Rather, the high rates of COVID-19 mortality within elder care facilities across North America and Europe may even increase the demand for home-based care of the elderly.

The COVID-19 lockdowns have potentially different effects upon MDWs depending in part upon whether or not they are live-in. The ability to work from home, and the job losses that accumulate as lockdowns continue, could reduce the willingness of households to hire or retain MDWs. Lockdowns can also increase the burden of care work that needs to be performed within the household. As we discuss in greater detail below, the work intensity of many live-in MDWs increased, as did their dependence upon their employers. For MDWs who are not living with their employers, lockdowns could mean an inability to work, and thus a loss of employment and income. These are MDW-specific impacts, in addition to the impact upon all migrant workers of being cut off from international travel. As a result, the specific design of mobility restrictions plays an important role in shaping outcomes for MDWs (Table 6.1).

The extent to which pre-existing systems of labor law and social protection include migrant workers matter greatly. Greater access to social protection programs, including subsidized healthcare, disproportionately helps MDWs, given that they are less likely to be covered by labor laws. But countries varied in the extent to which post-COVID relief programs specifically included migrants, in ways that did not always correlate with the wider socio-legal environment of democracy. The United States, for example, performed worse in this regard than some authoritarian states in the Middle East (Table 6.1).

Table 6.1. Graphical summary of Migrant-related COVID Responses, case study countries

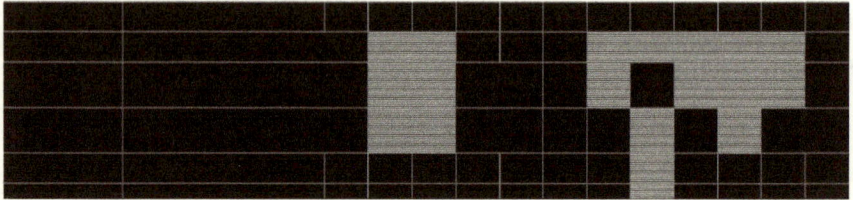

Black=Adequate, Stripes=Provisions exist but inconsistent, White=Inadequate/No provision
Source: Based on qualitative interviews, media searches and analysis of official social provisioning policies.

Host country advocacy and action also has a role to play. Remittance income is a critical source of expenditure and investment for receiving households in the South (Ratha et al., 2020). Remittances have helped recruit foreign exchange earnings for Southern governments in a neo-liberal world of low taxation and dollar denominated debt, with remittances from women migrants, including MDWs, being especially stable sources of foreign exchange. And yet, we found a few examples of host country governments mobilizing to provide direct or indirect support to MDWs. Instead, mobilization by MDWs themselves, with the support of migrant advocacy groups, turned out to be more significant.

In the host country analysis that follows, we investigate how these different factors, together with the underlying context of immigration laws, shaped the impact of this crisis upon the well-being of MDWs.

Host Country Analysis

In this section we draw on the key informant interviews as well as media searches and documentation of country-level immigration, social distancing and social protection policies (Gentilini et al., 2020). In investigating the impacts upon MDWs, we focused i) on the extent to which their well-being was considered in the design of travel restrictions; ii) their access to social protection both before and during COVID-19 lockdowns; and iii) the impact of host country interventions post-COVID-19, as summarized in Table 6.1.

Mobility Restrictions and Work

The most common national level response to COVID-19 in the period between February and May 2020 was the imposition of a lockdown. The Blavatnik School of Government, University of Oxford Stringency Index shows the variations in the strictness of lockdowns in the countries we studied (Hale et al., 2020). The index collates publicly available information on containment and closure policies, such as school closures and restrictions in movement, reporting a number between 1 and 100 to reflect the scale and depth of lockdown measures.

Countries imposed lockdowns at different points in time and with different degrees of harshness (Figure 6.1). As a consequence, migrants were caught between differential degrees of lockdowns in home and host countries. More stringent lockdowns included measures that were especially harmful to MDWs, including bans on international travel. Thus in the case of MDWs working in Hong Kong,

> *"those who had returned home for holidays were stranded. Some managed to come back [to Hong Kong] later on, but they had to submit to a 14 day quarantine. During quarantine, they didn't get wages. Migrant domestic workers have debts [due to paying for their own travel to the host countries] and they are mandated to live with their employers. [Hong Kong] made no arrangement for migrant domestic workers during their mandated quarantine and employers didn't allow them in, so many didn't know where to go, they got desperate, no one wanted them, and the government was never clear about where they should go." SME, Hong Kong.*

Others were trapped in destination countries. "Many of the people who would maybe want to go home cannot due to travel restrictions. For mixed immigration status families, they have been here on average 10-15 years, so going back to the home country is not a viable option." SME, US. Their mobility within the host-country was restricted and they were confined to employers' houses and places of work or to their communities. In Italy, for instance, during peak stringency all individuals were required to produce permits to enable them to be out on the streets. In Lebanon and Jordan, curfews were imposed at certain times with no exceptions.

SMEs shared that neighborhoods densely populated by migrants were disproportionately deprived of services and faced more severe lockdowns. Once confined to these neighborhoods migrant communities had more limited access to food, healthcare and other services than non-migrant neighborhoods (reported for Jordan, Lebanon, Kuwait, Singapore and parts of Spain and Italy).

Figure 6.1. Stringency Index over time, case study countries

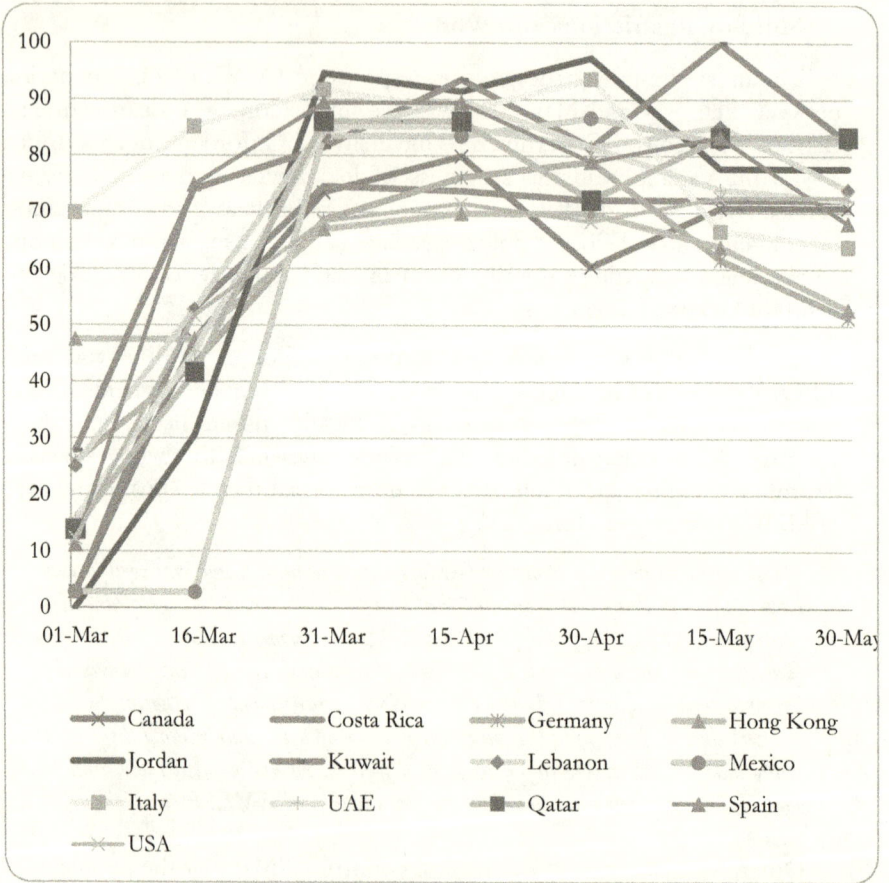

Source: https://covidtracker.bsg.ox.ac.uk/stringency-scatter; see Hale et al 2020 for explanation.

Many MDWs travel on sponsored visas linked to specific employers in host countries. These sponsorship visas mandate an exclusive relationship where the migrant either lives with the employer or works exclusively for them. Ostensibly, this link provides security for both the worker and employer. However, it also limits worker freedoms if the terms and conditions of employment are not favorable to the worker.

> *"Workers are not seeking healthcare because they are worried about being deported. Because their jobs and visas are tied to one employer, they are worried that if they do leave, they cannot come back to their jobs in the Middle East. We heard this directly from our migrant domestic network in Jordan." SME, Jordan.*

During COVID-19, this link caused a particular vulnerability, with employers abruptly working from home and no longer having the daily need for the worker. With a visa linked to one employer, migrants were in legal limbo – largely unprotected by emergency pandemic response measures, unable to look for new work, unable to qualify for protections like unemployment insurance, and unable to leave the country due to travel restrictions.

This reality underscores the intimate link between labor and migration policies: where countries did not extend visas and work permits for migrants, social distancing measures left many MDWs without jobs and without legal status in the host countries; some were expelled from their employers' houses and some have even been detained in government facilities.

Migrant domestic workers with multiple employers, were especially hurt in the US, Hong Kong, Jordan, Lebanon and in those countries where their migration status is linked to their employment status or where welfare and social assistance payments required migrants to present evidence of employment loss.

Conversely, mobility restrictions caused some employers to formalize their relationships with their workers so that they could continue in their employment, as in Italy where police strictly enforced checks of work permits including the name and number of the employer. "If the police stopped the person, they would be jailed. So employers have regularized contracts because of this fear of control that wasn't there prior to COVID." SME, International Agency.

Among live-in workers where employment loss did not lead to loss of shelter, SMEs reported a higher risk of MDWs being trapped in abusive employment relationships without wages or sufficient compensation (reports from Kuwait, Jordan, Hong Kong and Italy).

> *"The documented ones are not asking for emergency paid sick leave because they work for such small employers and the unequal power dynamic leaves them afraid for their jobs if they do so… Not having access to [personal protective equipment] has been a big issue for those continuing to work, especially because they cannot access emergency paid leave… Nannies who previously did not live in are in many cases being forced to become live-in or else will lose their jobs, their ability to renew visas." SME, US*

Sources reported that live-in MDWs in Jordan, Italy, and Lebanon were not getting paid, were unable to send remittances home, and were prohibited from leaving their work under the pretext of protecting the host family's health. In the US, many workers had no choice but to move in with their employers to shelter in place together or else lost the job entirely.

> *"Confinement with families means that the migrant domestic workers' rights depend*

entirely on the family. Some are reportedly not allowed rest days. Some are not even able to connect with [their own] families." SME, Middle East.

A few host countries provided amnesty to undocumented migrant workers (Kuwait) or regularized their status (Italy) as public health safety measures. Others are automatically extending visas to those who had a tourist or work visa (Costa Rica) or allowing workers to apply for extensions without having to return home (US). However, more often than not these provisions came about after a home country negotiated with a host country on behalf of migrants. In most cases, MDWs are fending for themselves in increasingly hostile environments to foreigners. Stories of migrants being deported further contributed to this fear, such as in the US where deportations increased over 6,000 in the month of March, or in Costa Rica, Hong Kong, Kuwait, and Jordan where all non-native migrants were told that if they returned home they would not be allowed back into the country.

Social Protection Access: Patchwork Reponses and Evidence of Exclusion

In many countries, MDWs who lost jobs were not eligible for income support, and yet those who remained working, some in very precarious conditions, continued to bolster systems of social protection and welfare provision they themselves could not access. Italy best exemplifies this tragic situation, where harsh mobility restrictions included requiring a permit in order to leave the house, domestic workers were excluded from income replacement schemes. Yet domestic workers were also declared essential workers – and were allowed to be mobile and given permits to work.

Host countries provide varying degrees of social protection for MDWs (Table 6.1). Canada has arguably the most robust system which pre-COVID-19 was estimated to cover about 99.8% of its population effectively (ILOSTAT 2020, Gentilini et al 2020). Anyone working in Canada who loses their employment because of COVID-19, but can prove that they were working, is entitled to a federal support program (channeled through employment insurance) and emergency unemployment insurance.

Costa Rica also has a well-developed social protection system, particularly for a middle-income country, which covered about 72% of its population (ILOSTAT 2020; Gentilini et al 2020). It has now implemented an emergency social protection measure that applies to domestic workers and even migrants, including monthly cash payments for three months that cover loss of work or reduction in hours.

"In Costa Rica, there were targeted measures such as the Protect Bonus which is a bonus for loss of work or reduction of working hours. It would apply to domestic

workers and even migrants, it is around $200 for three months and can be extended if necessary." SME, Costa Rica.

Other host countries include MDWs under the same legal protections that native-born workers enjoy (Hong Kong) or, if the paperwork is there, allow employers to contribute to social security and accumulate pensions and unemployment insurance (US). In the wake of COVID-19, Qatar is considering asking all the national banks to give MDWs an account for electronic salary payments. If this comes to pass, it could result in more formalization of work.

The unwillingness to extend healthcare to undocumented workers even in the midst of a pandemic starkly revealed the limitations of many formally democratic contexts. Thus in the US, "some money has been allocated to [federally qualified health centers] to cover testing for undocumented workers, but when there are not enough tests, what is the point?" SME, US. Interestingly, while few of the social protection measures put in place were targeted at migrant workers and MDWs in particular, some countries provided additional support to households regardless of residency status and provided financial transfers for caring for children and the elderly. Germany, Spain, Costa Rica and the US provided childcare-related transfers subsidies in recognition of the need to care for children. These measures may have enabled host countries to ensure that some MDWs retained their jobs.

The pandemic highlights the difficulties of enforcing workplace regulation of private households. Workers who apply for coverage under any existing provisions are the few who have internet access, sufficient knowledge of their rights, and access to the necessary documentation. Even where there are some protections, as in Costa Rica, employers may force workers to renounce their claims for additional benefits in exchange for corroborating unemployment. Workers are largely at the whim of their employers who may or may not continue to pay them while they shelter-in-place, putting them at risk of exposure to the virus or the police in order to look for work. Medical costs are often the responsibility of the employer, but the sponsorship system in many countries means workers are at the mercy of employers.

Inadequate Home Country Responses

Countries of origin with large migrant diaspora have responded to the pandemic in an un-coordinated fashion, with conflicting and confusing policies. Some governments appear to be seeking indemnity and actively refusing to help migrant workers in host countries. In Canada, one group of activists and academics reported that Jamaica had required outgoing migrants leaving on care visas to sign waivers that do not oblige them to be repatriated and cared for if they fall sick. "For example the Jamaican government is making migrants sign a waiver, stating that the Jamaican government does not have to look after them if they get sick in Canada." SME, Canada. In Costa Rica, primarily Nicaraguan migrants have had no support from their home country government. "In Costa Rica we have not seen interventions by Nicaragua. The case of Nicaragua is very dramatic... this is very worrying." SME, Costa Rica.

Very few countries of origin responded to the emergency by bringing MDWs home. Repatriation is hotly debated within home countries, largely centered around who pays for the flights and how and where migrants will be quarantined upon returning home. These constraints have led to stalemates, such as in Nepal where courts have ruled that the government must bring back all migrants, but the government has not made any steps toward this. In India, the government organized flights home but asked migrants to pay for them, two months into a lockdown that resulted in the loss of income for many of those migrants.

The Philippines and Bangladesh appear to be engaging with host country governments in some of the Gulf countries to support their migrant workers, but few flights had been made available for returning migrants and the responsibilities for payment remained unclear. The Filipino government did reach an agreement with the Kuwaiti authorities to implement amnesty for those workers who are or have become undocumented. The hope is that undocumented migrant workers will not be afraid to go to their embassies to register for financial assistance or to seek help to fly them back home. A few home countries sought to bring information to migrants: an emergency online portal (Sri Lanka in host countries), emergency phone lines (provided by consulates in Jordan), or free access to the Internet (negotiated in Qatar) for migrants to access health information and connect with embassies. Sri Lanka's online portal, *Contact Sri Lanka,* registered around 17,000 migrant workers by the end of April, over 6,000 of whom work in the Gulf. The Sri Lankan embassy in Kuwait was also making travel documents available online so that migrant workers do not need to apply for them in person.

Claims-making by Migrant Groups in Home and Host Countries

Without systematic or reliable help from home countries, migrants and migrant rights organizations have responded *ad hoc* to fill the gaps created by their exclusion from social protection systems. Migrants are organizing food drives for others unable to leave lockdown neighborhoods, creating cash relief funds, and working with civil society organizations to organize donations online. The biggest and most immediate impact has been in terms of provision of direct relief to MDWs in distress.

"MDWs have lost jobs, [it is a] crisis situation. Many have no food, no money,

no social protection, no health care, and they are also afraid to reveal their identities. We decided to spend our funds to set up a solidarity fund, to send our funds to affiliates. In the beginning we said we were not [a] humanitarian organization, but we changed our minds because the situation was so bad." SME, Hong Kong, talking about the situation in Singapore and parts of Asia.

"Before the virus, Lebanon was in economic crisis, since October they have had a massive devaluation, [the] financial crisis has affected everyone, wages were cut, a huge economic crisis, many migrant domestic workers lost jobs and now the virus is only making it so much worse. Luckily some non-governmental organizations (NGOs) in Lebanon work with us and have tried to give out cash and find shelters and organize local people to help them....drive them to work, offer collective transport, provide food and shelter. We are providing support as well, financially." SME, Hong Kong, speaking about the situation in Lebanon.

In home countries, some NGOs are also mobilizing to support returnees. In Bangladesh, BOMSA, a migrant rights NGO, created COVID-19 awareness-raising leaflets specifically for migrant domestic workers returning to Bangladesh from abroad. Members of BOMSA are distributing soap, disinfectant and other cleaning supplies, and encouraging workers to maintain social distance.

In the face of inadequate social protection systems, and COVID-19 responses that don´t take migrants and undocumented workers into account, many migrant rights organizations are also beginning to make claims on home and host country governments. One such alliance of organizations in Jordan is demanding that the government grant migrant workers legal residency during COVID-19, as many visas and work permits will expire during lockdown. The alliance is calling for the government to grant financial assistance to migrant workers, who have little or no pay but cannot return to their country of origin. The alliance also asks for safety gear for migrant workers still on the job.

Migrant organizing has also become virtual in the lockdowns. The domestic workers solidarity network in Jordan shares information about COVID-19 and its impact on workers in multiple languages on its Facebook page. Venezuelan immigrants in Costa Rica are organizing virtual migration and asylum workshops with immigration lawyers, NGOs and UN organizations. US advocates have leveraged online support resources including counseling, PPE use training, and know-your-rights training. SMS campaigns in Qatar provide MDWs and their employers with information about rights and protections.

Authoritarian contexts did constrain these responses in some ways. The SMEs we spoke to often requested anonymity due to the fear of reprisal, and the banning of unions created additional hurdles for organizers.

Nevertheless, claims-making did occur across these contexts, even if it took more informal forms.

"There is a network of migrant domestic workers in Jordan. They are not allowed to join unions in Jordan. They created a network of... migrant community leaders. These leaders share information about COVID-19 and have a Facebook page. All organizing is virtual." SME, North Africa Region.

Where the MDWs engage with unions and social movements in host countries, they necessarily articulate with a longer process of claims-making around labor rights, decent work, family reunification or pensions. Hence the claims-making will likely live on beyond the pandemic. If they are deported and their employment relations severed, MDWs as a whole will have less ability to continue to make claims in host countries. While the long-term impact of these mobilizations remains to be seen, their energy and urgency is undeniable.

Conclusions

COVID-19 has brought to the fore the critical role of care work undertaken by migrant domestic workers who are both essential and excluded workers—essential to social protection systems yet excluded from many rights and protections afforded other native workers. Ten years after the signing of Convention 189, decent work for domestic workers and particularly MDWs remains elusive. This crisis has thrown the exclusions and discrimination into sharp relief.

Stringent lockdowns, social distancing, and travel restrictions were imposed in many countries. Very stringent lockdowns without social protection left many migrants and particularly MDWs without employment and livelihoods, and others even more dependent upon their employers for shelter, as well as food and income, during the lockdowns. As well, migrant communities have been hit hard by COVID-19. To date, few home countries have attempted to bring migrants home and where they have, migrants have had to bear at least some costs.

Yet claims-making is occurring, even under these conditions. In many contexts, organizing has become virtual. NGOs and unions are working together to provide shelter, food, ensure access to information and channel assistance or demand host country governments react to abuses. Countries with more robust social protection systems and more inclusive migration regimes have responded better and more efficiently to the needs of MDWs in Canada, Costa Rica and Germany. With the plight of millions of women migrants in the balance, we surface the following recommendations from MDW groups and rights organizations:

Revisit the sponsorship system

COVID-19 puts the risks of this system into the starkest terms – tying employees to specific employers restricts MDWs freedoms of choice and puts them entirely at the whims of that employer. Migration and labor policy must uphold rights-based tenets that enshrine fundamental rights and freedoms such as decent work and the right to organize.

Social protections must include all migrants

COVID-19 heightens the vulnerabilities of undocumented migrants, many of whom currently have no choice but to overstay their visas and continue working in order to survive and to send remittances. Expanding social protections to all migrants regardless of immigration status or employment status is essential.

Formalize payment systems and wages and social security payments

All employers benefiting from state-sanctioned visas should be required to formalize wages and employment and provide verifiable wages and payments.

Prioritize human dignity in public health crises

COVID-19 underscores the truism that all health is public. There is no social benefit to only protecting some essential workers while implicitly or explicitly risking the lives of others based on migration or citizenship status, as this ultimately increases risks (either directly, through infection, or indirectly, through loss of access to provision of later) to overall public safety that are far costlier than preventive measures.

References

Altman, M. & K. Pannell (2012). "Policy Gaps and Theory Gaps: Women and Migrant Domestic Labor" *Feminist Economics*, 18:2: 291-315.

Boris, E. and M. Undén (2017). 'The Intimate Knows No Boundaries: Global Circuits of Domestic Worker Organizing" pp 245-268 in Michel Sonia, and Ito Peng I. eds. *Gender, Migration and the Work of Care: Gender, Migration and the Work of Care: A Multi-Scalar Approach to the Pacific Rim*. New York: Palgrave Macmillan.

Donato, K. and D. Gabaccia (2015). *Gender and International Migration*. Russell Sage Foundation. 2015.

Gentilini, U. et al. (2020). Social Protection and Jobs Responses to COVID-19: A Real-Time Review of Country Measures "Living paper" version 10, May 22, 2020. Retrieved from https://www.ugogentilini.net/wp-content/uploads/2020/05/Country-SP-COVID-responses_May22.pdf.

Hale, T. et al. (2020). "Variation in government responses to COVID-19 BSG-WP-2020/032 Version 5.0," April 2020, *BSG Working Paper Series*, University of Oxford.

ILO. 2016. Who Cares for the Carers? ILO, Geneva. Retrieved from s

ILOSTAT (2020). ILO Department of Labor Statistics. Retrieved from ILOSTAT.ilo.org, May 25, 2020.

IOM (2020). *World Migration Report 2020*. Geneva: International Organization for Migration.

Kontos, M. (2013). "Negotiating the Social Citizenship Rights of Migrant Domestic Workers: The Rights to Family Reunification and a Family Life in Policies and Debates. *Journal of Ethnic and Migration Studies* 39: 409-424.

Oliviera, G. (2017). "Caring for Your Children: How Mexican Immigrant Mothers Experience Care and the Ideals of Motherhood" pp 91-114, in Sonya Michel and Ito Peng (eds) *Gender, Migration, and the Work of Care: A Multi-Scalar Approach to the Pacific Rim*, Palgrave MacMillan.

Pérez Orozco, A. (2016). "Global Care Chains. Reshaping the Hidden Foundations of an Unsustainable Development Model," pp. 102-128 in Meghani, Zara (ed) *Women Migrant Workers, Ethical, Political and Legal Problems*, Routledge: New York and London.

Ratha, D. et al. (2020). "COVID-19 Crisis Through a Migration Lens" *Migration and Development Brief*, 32. KNOMAD, World Bank.

Varia, N. (2006). "Sanctioned Abuses: The Case of Migrant Domestic Workers. *Human Rights Brief* 14. 2006.

WHO (2017). *Women on the Move, Migration, Care Work and Health*. Geneva: World Health Organization.

CHAPTER 7

'UNWANTED BUT NEEDED' IN SOUTH AFRICA: POST PANDEMIC IMAGINATIONS ON BLACK IMMIGRANT ENTREPRENEURS OWNING SPAZA SHOPS

Sadhana Manik

Introduction

It is now widely accepted that post-apartheid, SA is a magnet given its political stability in Africa with a constitution underpinned by human rights. It has become an economic nucleus: being the second largest economy in Africa with a GDP of $348.8 billion and perceived by many Africans as a land of opportunity, thus attracting migrants from across the continent (Langalanga, 2019) and beyond. The Institute for Security Studies, (2018) however declared that "Migration in South Africa is a complex issue that is highly politicised and often volatile" and this volatility and its political and socio-economic armaments have been evident before and during the COVID-19 pandemic and which will influence its future. Many migrants are impacted upon by the country's policies and practices which are risk oriented, with the explicit aim of keeping prospective migrants (with the exception of highly skilled migrants) outside the country through securitization of the borders and numerous immigration deterring efforts (The Institute for Security Studies, 2018). For those who manage to cross the border into SA and are not highly skilled, their dreams are not easily achieved, as the literature (highlighting immigrants' experiences), policies and socio-economic practices landscape in South Africa attest to a track record of purposeful segregation, one that points to unwavering alienation and separation of foreigners from SA citizens in a multitude of ways oblivious and disregarding of immigrants' human rights. The risk lens taken by government extends to immigrants who are already resident within its borders and this sets the tone for a sustained anti-immigrant stance from politicians and government structures filtering all the way down to communities.

This chapter is focuses specifically on the plight of immigrant small/ micro business entrepreneurs (who are owners of 'spaza' shops in townships in post- apartheid South Africa) by offering up three 'imaginations' as post pandemic possibilities for the future of immigrant spaza shop owners. The theoretical construct of 'imaginations' is extrapolated from critical geopolitics where seminal author O'Tuathail (1996) makes reference to 'geopolitical imaginations.' Muller (2008: 323, 326) explains that it encapsulates "the imaginary spatial positioning of people, regions, states and the shifting boundaries that accompany this positioning." Polegkyi, (2020: 171) states that it is a way of 'visualizing the world and a country's place' therein. It has also been explained as a strategy that politicians use through media and technology to convey their specific ideas which can be perceived as propaganda (Ahmadypour, Hafeznia, Juneidi, 2010: 8-10). It is thus commonly understood that geopolitical imaginations are closely tied to discourses and geopolitical identities and this has relevance for immigrant entrepreneurs in South Africa. Therefore, in this chapter, my use of 'imaginations' refers to the nature of a post pandemic South Africa and the possible socio-economic and political positioning of immigrant spaza shop owners ('entrepreneurs' is uated interchangeably) therein.

However, before I embark on this, it's vital to trace the realities of the politics (policies and practices), socio-economic events and immigrant experiences pre COVID-19 and during the pandemic which sets the scene and provides a vivid backdrop for these three imaginations. I argue in this chapter that the 'auras' created about immigrant spaza shop owners find expression in public spheres and bolster the 'immigrant-as-a-criminal' discourse and other associated demeaning Black[1] immigrant discourses in SA society. The concept of 'aura' draws from Roy (2005) who writes extensively on the phenomenology of urban informality and how impressions (which she terms 'auras') can be textually established. In this chapter, the impressions created in policies and by government structures and politicians are highlighted as it could allow for the perpetuation of a xenophobic race based political and socio-economic agenda post the pandemic. The auras established and negative immigrant discourses could also curtail SA's revitalization of the economy and efforts at reaching its development goals post the pandemic.

I begin by illuminating the link in post-apartheid SA between unemployment and poverty amongst the native African population living in townships, entrepreneurship in the spaza shop sector and the arrival of immigrant entrepreneurs. This is followed by a discussion of who are the instruments of socio-economic and political anti-immigrant auras and discourses in SA. Pre pandemic immigrant experiences of xenophobia follows and the efforts to plunder and purge the townships of immigrant

---

[1] In South Africa, Black is an accepted term which refers to African, Indian, Coloured (mixed race) and Chinese populations who were previously disadvantaged during apartheid.

spaza shops during the pandemic. The chapter concludes with a presentation of the pandemic as a watershed moment with three post pandemic imaginations derived from key features of immigrant spaza shop entrepreneurs' experiences in SA.

Unemployment, Immigrant small and micro business Entrepreneurs and Spaza Shops

Post-apartheid South Africa (SA) has faced numerous challenges and a persisting one has been the increasing levels of unemployment especially amongst the majority African population. Across a 10 year period (2008–2018), the unemployment rate has continued to increase from 21,5% to almost 28,0% (Statistics SA, 2018). Mkoka (2012) revealed that the African population in South Africa, after apartheid did not have the necessary skills for formal employment given the socio-economic injustices of apartheid South Africa. Thus, the informal economy in democratic SA provided the opportunity for survival, an escape from poverty and unemployment (Fourie, 2018) more than a desire to be an entrepreneur.

The emergence and growth of spaza shops in township areas is an important step towards addressing poverty, reducing unemployment and developing the economy and character of township lifestyles. A spaza shop is explained as "a business operating in a section of an occupied residential home or in any other structure on a stand in a formal or informal township which is zoned for residential purposes and where people live permanently" (Ligthelm, 2008). Townships were designated living spaces according to race in apartheid South Africa, many of which have since become areas of poverty and strife. Spaza shop owners are thus seen as entrepreneurs in this context (Ngwenya, 2017; Tengeh and Mukwarami, 2017). Spaza shops were perceived as an innovative uniquely South African native business model in the informal economy. The South African government was keen to support native entrepreneurship in the informal economy given the need to address the imbalances of the past created by the previous regime's socio-economic engineering and therefore immigrants venturing into this sector were neither anticipated nor welcomed. There was a huge influx of African immigrants (from Zimbabwe, Cameroon, Nigeria, Senegal, Ethiopia, Somalia) between 2010 and 2015 into the spaza shop sector of the informal economy in townships (Tengeh, 2016) and this was followed by Indians (from Pakistan and Bangladesh) and some Chinese immigrant entrepreneurs (Lin, 2014; Willemse, 2014). African immigrant spaza shop owners currently dominate the spaza sector, exceeding the Bangladeshis and Pakistanis (Ngwenya, 2017)[2]. Presently, there are over 100 000 spaza shops in South Africa with

---

[2] There are no statistics or recent estimates of the Chinese immigrant owners of spaza shops although it is known that they don't dominate grocery retail but rather clothing retail.

between 70-85% of them being foreign owned (du Toit, 2020). Charman & Peterson (cited in Crush et al., 2015: 10) reveal how the township economy has been enhanced by immigrant shop owners in the "diversity of products, business activities and opportunities" on offer.

Despite, these advantages to the socio-economic spaces created by immigrant entrepreneurs, the distasteful 'aura' of immigrants being 'unwanted' is frequently painted in the media by politicians, state actors and citizens feeding and fattening the 'immigrant - as- a-criminal' discourse. This was evidenced in the political commentary and government policies and when conflicts arose between native and immigrant spaza shop owners. The spaza shop sector has become a contested space (Ngwenya, 2017). Immigrant ownership was perceived as a threat to the sustainability of native owned spaza shops and this resulted in the closure of those native owned businesses that were unable to compete with immigrant spaza shops' low pricing structures and allowances of grocery purchases on terms (Liedeman et al., 2013). This created a 'vacancy' for more immigrant owners of spaza shops to fill these gaps (Ngwenya, 2017).

The informal economy and institutional support were not significant in South Africa's policies and practices up to 2011 and the first major attempts at informal economy recognition appeared in national legislation: namely in The 2013 Licensing of Business Bill and the 2014 National Informal Business Upliftment Strategy (NIBUS), however the key focus here was on the reduction of immigrant participation and the promotion of native entreprenurship (Rogerson, 2016; Skinner, 2016). Skinner (2016) highlights how the roadmap for NIBUS implementation included the 'foreign trader challenge' (DTI 2014: 10, 31) and 'the prioritisation of support to South African businesses to support their competitiveness' (DSBD & ILO 2016: 19). Reference is made in NIBUS for the Department of Home Affairs to control the influx of foreigners (Skinner, 2016). Rogerson (2016) also draws attention to South Africa's 'pro developmental approach' to South African entrepreneurs in the informal economy and its 'anti- developmental approach to immigrant entrepreneurs'. Even the latest migration legislation, The White Paper on International Migration (2017) is anti-immigrant in its orientation (Zanker & Moyo, 2020). In addition, provinces in SA are expected to develop responses to the above national legislation and they appear to mimic the very same anti- immigrant entrepreneur stance (Skinner, 2016). The aura of the immigrant entrepreneur as being unwanted is deeply embedded into national and provincial documents.

There were the numerous strategies introduced by national government after 2010 to specifically augment native re-injection into the spaza shop sector (Tengeh & Mukwarami, 2017). The Small Business Traders Upliftment Project received a monetary boost of R 50 million and this was aimed at teaching business skills (Zulu, 2015). Additionally, immigrant small business owners were needed for a specific purpose in this government venture: their expertise to impart knowledge and skills to the native entrepreneurs. They were invited to speak by government, namely by the Minister of Small Business Development, in the hope of business knowledge transference to native spaza shop owners (Mbata, 2015). It is thus evident that they were needed as instruments to achieve a specific government objective of nurturing native entrepreneurs. Inadvertently, it is a recognition of the socio-economic value of immigrant small business entrepreneurs. A study of spaza shops in the township of Khayelitsha in Cape Town by Basardien et al (2014) found that immigrant entrepreneurs did have a higher score when compared to local entrepreneurs on four important indicators which are valuable for the development goals and enhancing SA's economy- namely entrepreneurial orientation, achievement, innovation, personal initiative and autonomy.

Despite these acknowledgements in research and the strategic manipulation of immigrant spaza shop sector by government, immigrant spaza shop entrepreneurs are frequently subject to heinous practices which emit auras of socio-economic intolerance perpetrated by politicians, state actors (such as the Department of Home Affairs' officials and police) and ordinary citizens. Here, the discourse of the 'immigrant spaza shop owner as a criminal' is blatantly evident and it is little wonder that there are repeated efforts from politicians and government to citizens to 'eradicate' immigrant entrepreneurs.

Instruments of socio-economic and political anti-immigrant auras and discourses

SA pre COVID-19 was replete with anti-immigrant socio-economic and political discourses which served as an indicator of SA as a violent country for immigrants (Tati, 2008). Neocosmos (2006:02) blames politicians and state actors for their contribution to xenophobia and the criminal discourse at community level declaring that in post-apartheid SA, "politicians and state institutions …in the making of a culture of xenophobia…. this has filtered down to the whole of society." Most pronounced is the 'immigrant entrepreneur as a criminal' discourse and there are numerous examples of this.

In 2012, the provincial Limpopo police commenced 'Operation Hardstick' which was supposed to be 'a crime fighting initiative' but it only targeted small immigrant owned businesses and not SA citizens (Crush, Chikanda & Skinner, 2015 :01). Crush et al (2015: 01) detail that in total, over 600 business operators had their goods confiscated, they were fined for not being in receipt of a trading permit and they were informed that foreigners cannot have businesses in SA. This incident led to a supreme court case in

2014, where judgement was ruled against the state and the Supreme Court declared, "one is left with the uneasy feeling that the stance adopted by the authorities in relation to the licensing of spaza shops and tuck shops was in order to induce foreign nationals who were destitute to leave our shores" (Supreme Court, 2014, 25).

Despite this victory by foreigners, Crush et al (2015, p. 2) declare that this is an 'endemic problem' in SA and not peculiar to one province arguing that there exists a smorgasbord of "regulatory and legal obstacles and the culture of police and official impunity that confront small immigrant businesses…throughout South Africa." A year later, 'Operation Cleansweep' in the city of Johannesburg in 2013, enacted similar behavior targeting 6000 immigrant shop owners and once again the Constitutional Court ruled in their favour. Crush et al (2015) have argued that immigrants in SA are denigrated to being 'unwanted parasites'. Apart from the aura of immigrants as being vermin being espoused above, another discourse created and perpetuated has been of 'immigrant entrepreneurs as non-compliant to regulations and destructive to development.' In 2013, the Deputy Minister of Trade and Industry, Minister Elizabeth Thabethe exclaimed at a small medium and micro enterprise summit (Jacaranda FM News, 10 October 2013) that immigrants were responsible for 'hurting development in townships and rural areas' as well. She stated, "The scourge of South Africans in townships selling and renting their businesses to foreigners unfortunately does not assist us as government in our efforts to support and grow these informal businesses … You still find many spaza shops with African names, but when you go in to buy you find your Mohammeds and most of them are not even registered." This discourse reared its head again during the pandemic and I revisit it after a brief discussion of community xenophobic violence in the townships.

Pre Pandemic Immigrant Experiences of Xenophobia

Post- apartheid SA townships (Tati, 2008; Mthombeni et al., 2014) and cities (Peberdy & Rogerson, 2002; Zanker and Moyo, 2020) have been core areas where Black immigrant small business entrepreneurs have chosen to start up their businesses believing that they will be able to grow and sustain themselves economically with ease in these densely populated areas. Unfortunately these very same areas are hotspots for outbreaks and the spread of xenophobia and currently, the corona virus which 'does not distinguish according to passport and citizenship" (Zanker & Moyo, 2020:01). From 1994 to August 2014 -excluding the 2008 widely spread xenophobic attacks, there were 228 documented incidents of violence perpetrated against migrants and refugee businesses and a 5 year slice from 2010 to 2014 shows the highest number of incidents (Crush et al., 2015).

It is interesting to note that the violence was initially perpetrated by the African population in SA targeting African immigrants and it gained its own nomenclature, Afrophobia, which Chigumadzi (2019) claims is growing. Over time as Indian small business entrepreneurs from Bangladesh and Pakistan opened businesses in urban areas and townships, the xenophobic violence has extended to Indians as well. Bond (2020) draws attention to the repeated violence which has not been addressed in SA as "… a series of brutal xenophobic attacks in 2008, 2010, 2015, 2017 and 2019, aimed at regional immigrants – including hundreds of owners of the tiny shops". It has been asserted that competition in the townships is the continued reason for xenophobia (Liedeman et. al., 2013; Hikam & Tengeh, 2016). The incidents of looting generally commences in urban centres such as Johannesburg and Durban (Beardsley, 2019; Crush & Ramachandran, 2014) then it spreads to other urban centres and townships. The crime is perceived as so extensive and repetitive (Northcote & Dodson, 2015, Chigumadzi, 2019) that immigrant shop owners live in fear (Gastrow and Amit, 2013) and others introduce innovative methods of business and personal protection. For example, Gumbo (2015) writes about spaza shop owners in the township of Soweto who have hidden doors and reinforced burglar guards. Chinese entrepreneurs also exposed corrupt police extorting money from them and similarly, Zimbabweans revealed bribing border officials to send remittances across to Zimbabwe. Collectively, immigrant spaza shop owners thus annually experience the looting of their shops, physical violence and intimidation, extortion and other forms of corruption, forced displacements of themselves and their families- and these experiences have endured pre COVID-19 and during the pandemic. Whilst SA citizens as individuals, business owners or government actors have been organized in their treatment of immigrant business owners, SA politicians have consistently and unfairly called it 'criminal elements' (Crush et al., 2015; Chigumadzi, 2019) in an effort to escape the responsibility to address these repeated heinous activities.

Pandemic Purging and Plundering of Immigrant Spaza Shops

When the pandemic struck SA, it was the first country in Africa to announce lockdown measures as a result of the coronavirus began spreading, resulting in infections and deaths. SA was lauded internationally for this step with stage 5 lockdown being declared from the 27 March 2020 (Zanker & Moyo, 2020) however, currently it has the second largest number of infections and death rate in Africa. The president also declared a state of disaster upon lockdown (instituting governance by the Disaster Management Act3). During the pandemic, xenophobia did not abate and immigrant

---

[3] Which caters to a maximum of three months within which the country can operate under such conditions

owners of spaza shops, had to bear the brunt of attempts at political purging coupled with communities plundering their shops, being threatened by mafia styled syndicates and experiencing police brutality and corruption.

For immigrant entrepreneurs in grocery retail, such as spaza shops, the pandemic was not a time to capitulate as they were deemed part of essential services, so grocery outlets could remain open but it spelt gloom for immigrant spaza shop owners who were suddenly excluded from trading without warning. The Minster of Small Business Development (sic), Khumbudzo Ntshavheni, caused an uproar two days before the commencement of the lockdown when she declared that only those spaza shops owned, managed and run by South Africans would be eligible to be opened during the lockdown (Githahu, 2020). The aura of exclusion and discrimination between immigrant and native owned spaza shops was revealed. This was immensely problematic from a social justice perspective which is a pillar of the SA constitution and there is no provision in any of the lockdown regulations for any differentiation between South African and immigrant-owned spaza shops, so there is no basis in law to target small businesses owned by immigrants, for closure. Researchers were quick to respond. Bond (2020) exclaimed, "the brutally xenophobic character of that policy" was evident in her declaration. Kavuro, of the Department of Public Law at Stellenbosch University, said: "Ntsheveni's approach fails to take into consideration the legal positions of foreign nationals who are holders of permanent resident permits, refugee status permit, asylum-seeker permit and business visas and who were, on top of all of these permits, issued licences to run small business." This heralded another blow for immigrant spaza shop owners as it is argued that they do not contribute to the formal unemployment insurance fund and neither were they eligible for a COVID-19 government business grant (Bond, 2020; Mokgabudi, 2020) as a result of business closure. The criteria for these grants included business owners needing to provide a company bank account, company registration documents and up to date tax payments and spaza shop owners have been identified as not being compliant in studies (Ngwenya, 2017). A week later, the decision was reversed and spaza shop owners and informal food traders without a permit were allowed to apply for a temporary permit. In the case of immigrant owners, they had to be a legal immigrants in receipt of a valid passport with a visa for work issued by the Department of Home Affairs. Asylum seekers should similarly be in receipt of a permit allowing work (Rajgopaul, 2020). Illegal immigrants were clearly excluded.

Currently, in communities, immigrant spaza shop owners are also not safe during the pandemic. Sizani (2020) reports on supposed protection being offered to immigrant shop owners after there were attacks on them. Investigations revealed that more than a 100 immigrant owners of spaza shops in Nelson Mandela Bay received letters from an organization called "Youth Against Crime" which comprise of unemployed youth. These letters suggest 'donations' to the organization to protect the shops against criminals. The aura of 'extortion' of immigrant owners of spaza shops is strong. Interestingly, the need for immigrant owned spaza shops are highlighted by the leader who acknowledges that the organization values spaza shops which offer the purchase of goods on credit so they are beneficial to the local community. This doesn't appear to be an isolated incident and the organization claims to protect Somali and Bangladesh immigrant spaza shop owners in Johannesburg, and also Mthatha, East London, and Komani in the Eastern Cape. It is thus evident that the organization is extorting money from immigrant spaza shop owners across the country. Interestingly, immigrant owners in Port Elizabeth tell of police who have also been targeting these stores. Mutandiro (2020) similarly reports on immigrant spaza shop owners in Diepsloot, Johannesburg complaining of police brutality (harassment, goods and money) in what police minister Bheki Cele is referring to as "crime stabilisation" after a policeman was killed by an immigrant. The aura of police corruption and brutality is again evident in these cases during the pandemic. The immigrant business owners have expressed fear and are reluctant to report the crimes although they have revealed the photographs and video footage as evidence to several news reporters. Once again the discourses of 'the immigrant entrepreneur as a criminal' as well as 'the immigrant succumbing to victimization out of fear' are articulated in respect of these immigrant spaza shop entrepreneurs.

The role of civil society organizations in holding government accountable is important in a stable democracy and The Centre for Human Rights at the University of Pretoria and the Centre for Applied Legal Studies (2020) articulated critical messages to government during the lockdown by commending "the South African government for ensuring that non-national spaza shop owners are not discriminated against." They further suggested "that the government strengthens regulations and undertake practical measures to protect these persons in order to ensure that their businesses are not affected by actions that amount to xenophobia, during and after the COVID-19 crisis" which serves as an alert to government to tread carefully post the pandemic.

In June 2020, SA was in stage 3 lockdown and it had not opened its borders to international travel and immigrant entrepreneurs of small businesses were expressing concerns for their health and future given numerous incidents: They complained of food insecurity as they were also discriminated (for not having a SA identity document) against when food was distributed and having had their shops looted, many have lost money and possessions. The plunge into poverty is illuminated by Madonsela (2020) who draws the president's attention to corruption in the delivery of food parcels. Mardia (2020) interviewed Dr Abdul Karim Elgoni, the chairperson of the African Diaspora Forum, who also explained that he had "numerous requests for assistance from desperate people who want to return to the lands of their birth. He also raised concerns over the lack of interest in the plight of migrants, asylum seekers and refugees from their embassies in South Africa." It is clearly evident that immigrant spaza shop owners are being pushed to the fringes of society during the pandemic and are reaching disproportionate levels of poverty whilst being forced to remain within the borders of South Africa.

So what are the possible post pandemic imaginations for immigrant owners of spaza shops in South Africa given the above discussions.

The COVID-19 Pandemic as a Watershed Moment

I present three distinct imaginations that are generated from the above discussion. The first 2 imaginations presented are negative, being deeply hinged on socio-economic and political behavior emanating from the auras and discourses that that were evident pre COVID-19 and which also revealed itself during COVID-19. The third imagination provides a positive outlook drawing on critique pre and during COVID-19 from multiple platforms. These imaginations are also influenced by the articulations and case study experiences expressed at two Columbia University webinars on COVID-19 where the audience was urged to take cognizance that COVID-19 meant that " we are at a cross roads" and that the road now taken can fuel the inequalities." It is for this reason that I present this watershed moment where SA must carefully choose the trajectory to be followed during the easing up of the stages (alert levels) in the lockdown as weekly there is legislation being promulgated as guidance to open up the economy. However, South Africa does need to tread carefully as 2 June 2020 heralded a landmark case against government when the East Gauteng High Court ruled that stage (alert level) 3 and 4 lockdown regulations were 'invalid and unconstitutional' and government needed to revise these within two weeks. Government later announced on the 4 June that it would be appealing the decision. What is revealed here is the value of the law of the land, the constitution of SA for decision-making post the pandemic, in terms of equality, accountability and social justice.

Post Pandemic Imaginations

Imagination 1: In this scenario, securitization and risk strategies to supposedly protect citizens continue with an eclipsing of the needs of immigrants. There are two major impact strands, namely that immigrant spaza shop owners' socio-economic and political struggles continue. It has been documented pre COVID-19 that in general immigrant small business owners face "economic challenges including a lack of access to financial services… start up capital and on going credit… limited access to debt finance from commercial banks" etc. (Crush et al, 2015: 5) and despite their need for credit, when they do apply, they are generally refused. This will not abate. They rely on loans derived from their social networks which will now be difficult as COVID-19 is a global pandemic and everyone is cash strapped with lockdowns having deepened the vulnerability of many families. Thus with more than two months of COVID-19 strife (with immigrant spaza shop owners facing political wrath, police extortion and corruption and community looting and extortion) in South Africa, it will be an uphill battle for immigrant spaza shops to survive. In this imagination, the current COVID-19 status quo prevails with the perpetuation of these antagonistic attitudes and xenophobic behavior supported by policies, politicians, communities and government structures. The anti-immigrant auras (aligning immigrants to the unwanted persist: criminal, parasites, vermin) and discourses such as the 'immigrant entrepreneur as a criminal' and 'immigrant entrepreneurs as non-compliant to regulations and destructive to development', remain entrenched in all aspects of socio-economic and political life.

When The Small Business Development Minister Khumbudzo Ntshavheni showed 'brazen' xenophobia (Bond, 2020) during COVID-19, the battle to survive for immigrant small business entrepreneurs in South Africa was tested. Indeed, there will be activists (such as Thuli Madonsela) and civil society organizations (such as The Centre for Human Rights) with a strong law and social justice underpinning which will use public platforms and the structures in place (such as The Human Rights Commission and the Constitutional Court) to ensure that the social protection of citizens and immigrants endure and that human rights abuses do not prevail as the order of the day.

Imagination 2: In this secenario, SA sets the pace for regressive measures with COVID-19 being used as an excuse to embed more protectionist armaments in multiple ways, discriminating between us (citizens) and them (immigrants), heightening the socio-economic and political auras of immigrant entrepreneurs being 'unwanted' using metaphors of parasites and vermin accompanied by negative discourses of immigrant entrepreneurs as criminals and non-compliant to regulations and destructive to development. During the various stages of lockdown in SA, the social protections of immigrants are being eroded, leaving these entrepreneurs vulnerable in the host country and unable to return to their home country. In this imagination, "Purge South Africa of the Immigrant" becomes the dominant discourse with more restrictive policies being promulgated to protect citizens and job reservations and entrench segregation based on the nature of citizenship. A looming example of this is already forming through an organization called The African Transformation movement (ATM) which has "presented a post covid-19 economic recovery plan, that if adopted would see South Africans claiming back all the sectors that are perceived to be unfairly dominated by foreigners" (Mavusa, 2020) and this will definitely extend to immigrant owned spaza shop owners who have become a thorn to government and native spaza shops owners over the years. Vuyo Zungula, the leader declared that "the government must pass a law similar to what other countries are doing to ringfence the informal economy for South Africans." In a plan, titled 'Putting South Africa First" which he has submitted to government, he highlights that other African countries like Nigeria, Ethiopia and Ghana have already set the bar with legislation that exclude immigrants from certain sectors of economy. This is not new, as numerous countries in Africa, pre COVID-19 have immigration governance policies based on strict securitization measures which deter migration, similar to South Africa. The ideal of the African visa, allowing free movement of persons as envisaged in the AU Agenda 2063, (including immigrant entrepreneurs) which was delayed in implementation will disappear into the horizon amidst the enforcement of insular goals post the pandemic. This imagination will see SA's economy also plunge with reducing investment by immigrant spaza shop owners -as it has already contracted significantly currently occupying below junk status, with regional cooperation and numerous regional cooperation goals set in the AU agenda 2063 being greatly delayed.

Imagination 3: In this scenario, SA learns from the harsh lessons from the past, takes guidance from local heroes and it begins to bake in fruitful local and geopolitical endeavours regarding legislation and relationships with a positive ripple effect for immigrant spaza shop owners. Geopolitically, the enhancement of relationships with other countries in the continent features in a drive to reinvest in the AU's 2063 vision which starts becoming a priority. SA invests in regional and also global compacts and embarks on harnessing the opportunities created by COVID-19 to propel the economy especially the informal economy, towards real growth in climbing out of 'below junk' economic status.

Locally, the state begins to propagate positivity for immigrants and citizens alike because it has long been recognized as a key instrument in repeated incidents of xenophobia in SA (Tati, 2008). The post pandemic guidance comes from local and global COVID-19 heroes. South Africa's previous much loved and revered public protector Thuli Madonsela,4(2020)

---

[4] Now currently the Law Trust Chair at the University of Stellenbosch, South Africa.

articulated the challenges presented in the lockdown around 'social justice and reasonableness' which are strongly embedded in the Constitution of SA and these begin to guide plans for a post pandemic future. The constitution comes to the fore in all decision-making. Madonsela's (2020) utterances that the equality clause underpinned by social justice concerns in the constitution demands that no one in society must be "unjustly and unfairly excluded from opportunities, resources, benefits and privileges " become a guiding principle. Madonsela in a letter to the president on the 5 June 2020 asked the question: "How long will the cry of the young people in villages and townships – whose self- employment has ground to a halt, their unregistered businesses ineligible for loans and salary relief- go unheard?" This statement becomes a beacon serving as a reminder to tap the potential of all who live within its borders, especially village and township entrepreneurs and the young. Currently, unemployment which was 29.1% in the 3rd quarter of 2019 is the highest amongst SA's youthful population and in this imagination, the youth are employed in projects to register immigrant businesses such as spaza shops and ensure their compliance with business regulations and this then contributes to revenue and the economic development of SA.

Big business in SA has already committed a billion rands as a COVID-19 grant for small businesses and in this imagination, government engages in public private partnerships with large businesses to nurture and support small businesses such as spaza shops. Immigrant small business owners are clearly needed in SA for their socio-economic value and this recognition by government is translated into proactive opportunities and projects for knowledge and skills transfer for all budding entrepreneurs regardless of citizenship. The idea is to reignite the township spaza shop economy for all entrepreneurs, not sow divisions between immigrants and natives. South Africa follows Italy's lead in calling 'no one must be left behind.' A step in the right direction comes from a country driven to its knees during COVID-19, with Italy regularizing its immigrants and this propels SA to embark on similar measures to regularize its immigrants as it has already done with Zimbabwean immigrants.

Conclusions

Discussions at a recent webinar (Columbia University, 29 May 2020) warned that the lessons we are learning from COVID-19 are coming 'fast and furious' and that economics is the first priority in a post pandemic world. For numerous years, the hostility towards immigrant owned spaza shop entrepreneurs in the informal sector of the economy from the upper echelons, namely politicians and government spiraling all the way down to grass roots level has created a toxic environment in SA. The auras and discourses created by national policies and politicians which ripple down government structures to SA citizens, are of immigrant spaza shop entrepreneurs as being unwanted despite them being needed to grow the economy and to develop South African entrepreneurs. State actors such as the police are complicit in extortion in some instances and in others they fail to protect immigrant spaza shop entrepreneurs. Spaza shops are the life blood of the township informal economy in South Africa and with the majority of spaza shops being owned by foreigners, anti-immigrant policies and practices threaten the continued existence and growth of the spaza shop sector, which contributes to poverty alleviation and a reduction in unemployment (immigrant spaza shops are known to employ local South Africans as well). Spaza shops have a distinct contribution to make to the socio-economic development of SA (Mukwarami et al, 2018) and this should not be undermined by separatist policies and planning that distinguish owners on the basis of citizenship. Crush et al (2015) warn of a dearth of imaginative policy construction on the informal economy and the role of migrants.

Most importantly, History lays bare the details of how immigrants such as miners have built the formal economy of the country and more recently that immigrants have contributed a significant role in having shaped the informal township economy and creating entrepreneurial extensions. However their value goes unrecognised in SA (Crush, Chikanda and Skinner, 2015). The Centre for Human Rights, University of Pretoria, and the Centre for Applied Legal Studies (2020) has also reminded government during the COVID-19 pandemic of its commitment to non-discrimination contained in the National Action Plan to Combat Racism, Racial Discrimination, Xenophobia and Related Intolerances. The above is a clarion call for change and a need to be proactive.

The late Nelson Mandela claimed that South Africa is for all who live in it...clearly this was not the case pre and during the COVID-19 pandemic but it is perhaps the most appropriate time to make the necessary changes socio-economically and politically for an all-inclusive country regardless of citizenship, as envisaged by a man who spent 27 years in prison fighting for the freedom of all people in SA regardless of race or any other intersectional variable. Across the world, the establishment and growth of small businesses by immigrants is lauded in host countries for immigrants' socio-economic contributions (such as job creation and filling gaps in the market) but democratic South Africa has become one of the few exceptions. The pandemic has highlighted SA's erosion of its commitment to Human Rights and a side stepping of the African Union's (2019) thrust for regional unity and cooperation.

The aftermath of COVID-19 presents the opportunity, for government to invest in the informal economy, to harness immigrant spaza shop entrepreneurs who are being purposefully excluded and to build regional and global compacts to strengthen her foothold in Africa and the world through meaningful legislation that seeks to liberate and affirm immigrant entrepreneurs rather than eradicate them.

References

African Union. (2019). The Revised Migration Policy for Africa and Plan of Action (2018-2027). Addis Ababa: African Union.

Ahmadypour, Z., Hafeznia, M R., Juneidi, R. (2010). "Representing Imaginary Enemy: A Geopolitical Discourse". Geopolitics Quarterly, 6 (4): 7-40.

Bank, L. (2020). Covid-19 reveals migration links in South Africa's human economy. The Daily Maverick. Available at https://www.dailymaverick.co.za/article/2020-05-17-covid-19-reveals-migration-links-in-south-africas-human-economy/.17 May 2020.

Basardien, F., Parker, H., Bayat, M., Frederick, C and Sulaiman, A. (2014). "Entrepreneurial Orientation of Spaza shop Entrepreneurs in Khayelitsha". Singaporean Journal of Business Economics and Management Studies, 2: 45-61.

Beardsley, S. (2019). Migrant shop-owners fear more violence in South Africa. 2 Oct 2019. Available at https://www.dw.com/en/migrant-shop-owners-fear-more-violence-in-south-africa/av-50684852

Bond, P. (2020). Covid-19 attacks the down-and-out in ultra-unequal South Africa. 30 March 2020.Available at http://www.europe-solidaire.org/spip.php?article52739.

BusinessTech, 2020. South Africa's Lockdown Regulations are Invalid and Unconstitutional. Available at https://businesstech.co.za/news/government/404 291/south-africas-lockdown-regulations-are-invalid-and-unconstitutional-high-court/

Charman, A and Peterson, L. (2015). "A transnational space of business: the informal economy of Ivory Park, Johannesburg". In: Crush, J., Chikanda, A and C. Skinner (eds.) Mean Streets: Migration, Xenophobia and Informality in South Africa. Waterloo: South African Migration Project (SAMP).

Chigumadzi, P. (2019). Afrophobia is growing in South Africa. Why? Its leaders are feeding it. African Arguments. Available at https://africanarguments.org/2019/10/08/afrophobia-is-growing-in-south-africa-why-its-leaders-are-feeding-it/

COVID-19 Response: News, analysis and resources. https://www.tralac.org/news/article/14477-covid-19-resources-page.html

Crush, J., Chikanda, A and Skinner, C. (2015). "Migrant Entrepreneurship and informality in SA cities". In: Crush, J., Chikanda, A and C. Skinner (eds.) Mean Streets: Migration, Xenophobia and Informality in South Africa. Waterloo: South African Migration Project (SAMP).

Crush, J and Ramachandran, S. (2014). Xenophobic Violence in South Africa: Denialism, Minimalism, Realism. Migration Policy Series 66. Cape Town: South African Migration Project.

Department of Small Business Development & International Labour Office (DSBD & ILO). (2016). Provincial and local level roadmap to give effect to the national informal business upliftment strategy. Policy memo. Pretoria: DSBD

Department of Trade and Industry DTI. (2014).The National Informal Business Upliftment strategy (NIBUS). Policy memo. Pretoria: DTI

Du Toit, A. (2020). South Africa's spaza shops: how regulatory avoidance harms informal workers. The Conversation. Available at: http://theconversation.com/south-africas-spaza-shops-howregulatory-avoidance-harms-informal-workers-130837

Fourie, F. (ed).(2018). The South African Informal Sector: Creating Jobs, Reducing Poverty. Boulder: Lynne Rienner Publishers

Gastrow, V and Amit, R. (2013). Somalinomics: A Case Study on The economic Dimensions of Somali Informal trade in the Western Cape. Johannesburg: University of Witwatersrand African Centre for Migration and Society.

Githahu, M. (2020). Call for clarity on spaza shops during Covid-19 lockdown. Cape Argus News. Available at https://www.iol.co.za/capeargus/news/call-for-clarity-on-spaza-shops-during-covid-19-lockdown-45856999 . 31 March 2020.

Gumbo, T. (2015). "Resilience and Innovation: Migrant Spaza Shop entrepreneurs in Soweto, Johannesburg". In: Crush, J., Chikanda, A and C. Skinner (eds.) Mean Streets: Migration, Xenophobia and Informality in South Africa. Waterloo: South African Migration Project (SAMP).

Hikam, A and Tengeh, R.K. (2016). "Drivers of the perceived differences between Somali and native entrepreneurs in South African townships". Environmental Economics, 7(4): 102-110.

Institute for Security Studies. (2018). *Keep them Out-Costs of South Africa's Migration Policy.* ISS Seminar in Pretoria. 25 October 2018.Available at https://issafrica.org/events/keep-them-out-costs-of-south-africas-migration-policy.

Langalanga, A. (2019). A Tale of Two Continents: Comparing Migration Experiences in South Africa & Germany. Occasional Paper 296, Johannesburg: South African Institute of International Affairs.

Liedeman, R., Charman, A., Piper, L., & Petersen, L. (2013). Why are foreign-run spaza shops more successful? The rapidly changing spaza sector in South Africa. Available at www.econ3x3.org./article/why-are-foreign-run-spaza- shops-more-successful-rapidly-changing-spaza-secto r-south-africa.

Ligthelm, A.A. (2008). "A targeted approach to informal business development: the entrepreneurial route". Development Southern Africa, 25(4): 367–382.

Lin, E. (2014). "Big Fish in a small Pond: Chines Migrant shopkeepers in South Africa". International Migration Review", 48: 181-215.

Madonsela, T. (2020). An Open Letter to Cyril Ramaphosa. Business Live. Available at https://www.businesslive.co.za/fm/opinion/protected-space/2020-06-04-thuli-madonsela-an-open-letter-to-cyril-ramaphosa/

Mardia, T. (2020). 'It's been very hard; trying to eat and to survive' - a migrant's cry for help. 5 May 2020. Available at https://www.news24.com/SouthAfrica/News/its-been-very-hard-trying-to-eat-and-to-survive-a-migrants-cry-for-help-20200505.

Mavusa, S. (2020). ATM seeks to prohibit foreigners from certain jobs. IOL News. https://www.iol.co.za/news/politics/atm-seeks-to-prohibit-foreigners-from-certain-jobs-48454036. 24 May 2020.

Mbatha, A. (2015). "African Minister says Foreigners Must Share Trade Secrets." Bloomberg. Available at http://www.bloomberg.com/ news/articles/2015-01-28/s-africa-minister-says-Non South Africans-must-share-to-avoid-looting.

Mkoka, S. (2012). "Towards integrated youth development". My Youth My Future Journal, 1 (1): 2-103.

Mokgabudi, L. (2020). Spaza and Informal trade are excluded from COVID-19 relief efforts in South Africa. 16 April 2020. Available at https://bfaglobal.com/insight-type/blogs/spaza-shops-covid-relief-africa/.

Mthombeni, D., Anim, F. and Nkonki- Mandleni, B. (2014). "Factors that contribute to vegetable Sales by Hawkers in Limpopo". South Africa. Journal of Agricultural Science, 61: 197-204.

Muller, M. (2008). "Reconsidering the concept of discourse for the field of critical geopolitics: Towards discourse as language and practice". Political Geography, (27) 322-338.

Mutandiro, K. (2020). Ethiopian shop owners in Diepsloot say police are stealing their goods and cash during raids. Ground Up. 9 March 2020.Available at https://www.dailymaverick.co.za/article/2020-03-09-ethiopian-shop-owners-in-diepsloot-say-police-are-stealing-their-goods-and-cash-during-raids/.

Neocosmos, M. (2006). "From 'Foreign Natives' to 'Native Foreigners': Explaining Xenophobia in post-apartheid South Africa". Dakar: Council for the Development of Social Science Research in Africa.

Northcote, M and Dodsen, B. (2015). "Refugees and Asylum Seekers in Cape Town's Informal Economy". In: Crush, J., Chikanda, A and C. Skinner (eds.) Mean Streets: Migration, Xenophobia and Informality in South Africa. Waterloo: South African Migration Project (SAMP).

Ngwenya K. (2017). Somali immigrants and social capital formation: A case study of spaza shops in the Johannesburg township of Cosmo City. Unpublished Sociology Masters Thesis, University of South Africa, Johannesburg.

O.Tuathail, G. (1996). The Politics of writing Global Space. Minneapolis: University of Minnesota Press

Peberdy, S and Rogerson, C. (2002). "Transnationalism and South African Entrepreneurs in South Africa's SMME economy". In: J. Crush and D. MacDonald (eds.) Transnationalism and New African Immigration to South Africa. Toronto: South African Migration Project (SAMP).

Polegkyi, O. (2020). "Regional Cooperation in Ukrainian and Polish and Security Discourse." In: O. Bogdanova and A. Makarychev (eds.) Baltic-Black Sea Regionalisms: Patchworks and Networks at Europe's Eastern Margins, Cham: Springer.

Rajgopaul, D. (202). Government to allow small businesses and spaza shops to operate during lockdown. IOL Business News. 7 April. Available at https://www.iol.co.za/business-report/companies/government-to-allow-small-businesses-and-spaza-shops-to-operate-during-lockdown-46370673

Rogerson, C. (2004). "The Impact of the South African Government's SMME programme: A ten year Review (1994-2003)." Development Southern Africa, 21 (5): 765-784.

Rogerson, C. (2016). "South Africa's informal economy: Reframing debates in national policy". Local Economy, 31(1-2): 172–186.

Roy, A. (2005). "Urban Informality: Towards an epistemology of Planning". Journal of the American Planning Association. 71 (2): 147-158.

Sizani, M. (2020). Immigrant spaza shop owners asked for "donations" to protect them from criminals. Ground Up. 20 May 2020. Available at https://www.groundup.org.za/article/immigrant-spaza-shop-owners-approached-donations-protect-them-criminals/.

Skinner, C. (2018). "Informal Sector Policy and Legislation in South Africa: Repression, Omission and Ambiguity". In F. Fourie (ed). The South African Informal Sector: Creating Jobs, Reducing Poverty. Boulder: Lynne Rienner Publishers.

Statistics South Africa. (2019). Who is most likely to be affected by long term Unemployment. Available at http://www.statssa.gov.za/?p=11688

Supreme Court of Appeal. (2014). Somali Association of South Africa and Others versus Limpopo Department of Economic Development, Environment and Tourism and Others (48/2014).

Tati, G. (2008). "The Immigration Issues in the Post- Apartheid South Africa: Discourses, Policies and Social Repercussions", Geopolitics and Populations, 3: 423-440.

Tengeh, R.K. (2016). "Entrepreneurial Resilience: The case of Somali grocery shop owners in a South African township". Problems and Perspectives in Management, 14(4-1): 73-81.

Tengeh, R.K. and Mukwarami, J. (2017). "The Growth Challenges of Native-owned Spaza Shops in Selected Townships in South Africa". International Journal of Applied Business and Economic Research, 15 (22): 61-74.

University of Columbia. (2020). *COVID-19 Webinars- 08 and 29 May.* Held by Open

Foundations Society and Columbia University according to Chatham House Rules.

University of Pretoria News. (2020). Centre for Human Rights Statement on the plight of migrants in South Africa during COVID-19. 15 April 2020.Available at https://www.up.ac.za/news/post_2887872-chr-statement-on-the-plight-of-migrants-in-south-africa-during-covid-19.

Zanker, FL and Moyo, K. (2020). "The Corona Virus and Migration Governance in South Africa: Business As Usual?" Africa Spectrum, 1-13.

Zulu, L. (2015). Minister of Small Business Development, Small Business Development Budget Vote 2015/16). South African Government. Available at http://www.gov.za/speeches/minister-lindiwe-zulu-small-business-development-dept-   budget-vote-201516-20-may-2015-0000

CHAPTER 8

LABOUR MARKET AND MIGRATION OUTCOMES OF THE COVID-19 OUTBREAK IN MEXICO

Carla Pederzini Villarreal and Liliana Meza González

Employment and Migration in Mexico in times of COVID

One of the main results of the health crisis caused by the expansion of the coronavirus in Mexico is the plunge of the economic activity and the consequent reduction in employment. The pandemic adds to the negative performance that both the economy and the employment rate had been showing in the country. In January 2020, before the first COVID case, ILO had already estimated an increase in the unemployment rate in the country in 2020 and 2021. On the other hand, economic activity fell in Mexico -0.1 in 2019, which shows that Mexico was experiencing a recession before the pandemic onset.

The fiscal system in Mexico has favoured firms with low efficiency, fostering low productivity in the Mexican economy (Levy, 2018) and Levy and López-Calva (2017). On the other hand, due to an increase in the relative supply of highly educated workers, returns to education have fallen in the country (Campos, Esquivel and Lustig, 2016), leading to the argument that the Mexican labour force is overeducated and does not respond to the needs of the productive structure. Furthermore, the work by Meza and Rodríguez (2020) finds that investment in cutting-edge technology has been postponed in the country due to the low cost of labour. In this context, the fact that robots and digital applications could substitute workers due to the pandemic could mean an increase in labour productivity. However, at a cost of a higher unemployment rate.

Following the spread of the virus in Mexico, measures commending social distancing to minimize contagion have been taken. On March 23, the Mexican government suspended classes; the meetings of more than 100 people were banned and work activities that involved social mobilization were restricted. The main motivation to implement these measures was to ensure that the Health System could maintain the capacity to assist patients in need of medical care and ensure that the mortality rate did not skyrocket.

However, unlike some other nations, Mexico has not offered a large stimulus package to support its economy. The few actions taken so far include over a million microloans of about $1,000 (US dollars) to tiny businesses in both the informal and formal sectors. According to experts, this program will barely make a difference in a sector where some 30 million people work.

Compared to previous economic recessions in Mexico, the present crisis has impacted employment more severely. As a consequence of isolation measures, many companies have been forced to stop operating due to the substantial drop in the demand for their products or services, while others have reorganized to, as far as possible, carry out their operations remotely.

INEGI (Instituto Nacional de Estadística y Geografía) carried out a new employment survey based on interviews by telephone (ETOE) in order to temporarily substitute the national employment and occupation survey (ENOE) carried out every quarter. Even though, due to its smaller sample size, ETOE is not fully comparable with ENOE, it is a reliable source of information about the Mexican labour market. According to the ETOE data, the occupied population in Mexico decreased by 12.5 million between March and April 2020. Most of the impact occurred among informal workers, which fell from 31 million to 20.7 million. Formal workers went from 24.7 to 22.6 million, a considerable but less shocking decrease. Among the occupied population, the number of those who have the need and availability to offer more working time than their current occupation demands from them, rose from 5.1 million in March 2020 to 11 million (25.4% of the occupied population) in April 2020 (INEGI, 2020).

According to our own calculations, all working age groups experienced a substantial reduction in economic participation in April 2020 when we compare to April 2019, as shown in Figure 8.1.

However, when we look at economic participation by educational level (Figure 8.2), we find that workers with higher educational levels were able to keep their jobs during the pandemic, especially those with graduate studies. On the other hand, the less educated groups were the most affected.

Isolation measures cause less demand for labour and, most likely, the replacement of workers by robots and digital applications, a situation in which unskilled workers turn out to be the most affected. Highly qualified workers, on the other hand, show greater complementarity with technology; therefore, it is more likely that they will keep their jobs during and after the pandemic. These workers can have better conditions of isolation, because they can work remotely. Hence, in general, in the Mexican economy, low-skilled workers are the most disturbed by social distancing.

Figure 8.1. Participation in Economic Activty by Sex and Age Group (April 2019-April 2020)

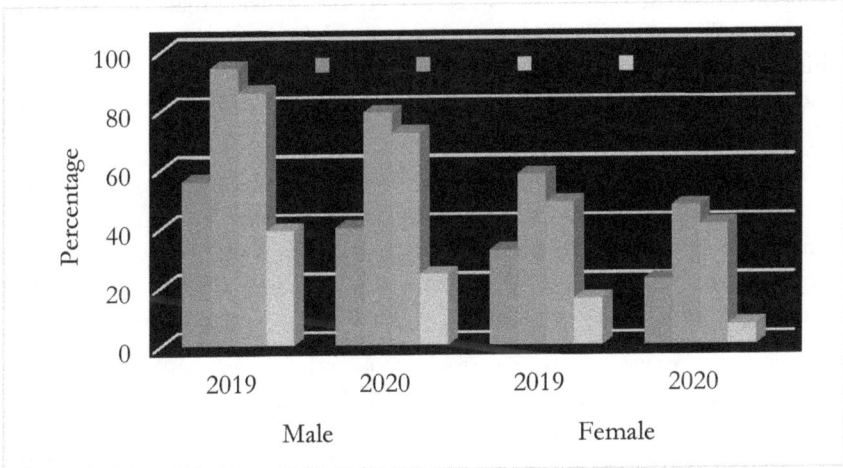

Figure 8.2. Participation in Economic Activty by Sex and Educational Level(April 2019-April 2020)

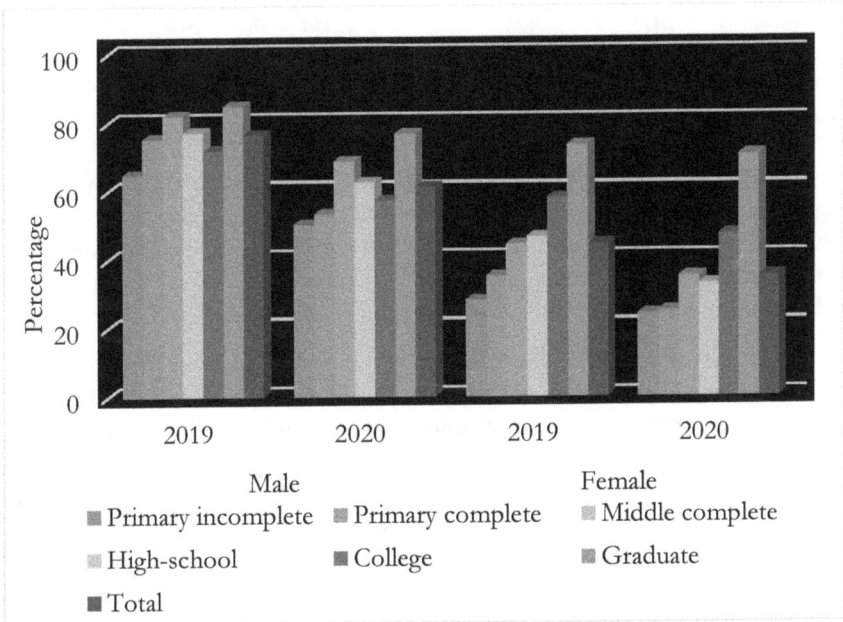

In relation to women's employment, the fact that their work is more complementary to technology could cause them to be less affected in relative terms. However, it has been found that, with social distancing, women are absorbing a higher burden of domestic work, as well as caring for children who are not attending school. In general, the outbreak experience means that women's domestic burden becomes exacerbated as well, making their share of household responsibilities even heavier, while they also work full time. This increased relative burden may lead to a drop in female productivity that might offset the positive effect of increased complementarity with technology.

Our comparison over the same period of the population not economically active and available for work, a normally highly feminized group, shows that female participation drops considerably as a result of the measures taken to fight the pandemic (Table 8.1). This result indicates a much higher male tendency to join the non-economically active and available for work group.

Table 8.1: Female partipation (%) in Population not economically active and available for work by Educational Level and Age Group

Educational Level	April 2019					April 2020				
	Age Group					Age Group				
	14-24	25-44	45-64	65 +	Total	14-24	25-44	45-64	65 +	Total
Primary incomplete	64.5	85.4	85.7	55.1	68.0	56.4	83.2	35.4	30.6	42.7
Primary complete	52.2	92.1	87.1	53.5	73.3	51.4	63.4	54.6	54.8	57.4
Middle School	61.6	91.0	80.8	34.8	75.2	56.1	73.4	56.7	44.1	64.1
High-school	54.4	89.0	72.3	52.2	63.9	45.7	57.7	54.4	58.0	53.3
College	55.4	62.0	70.1	17.5	57.9	37.4	48.9	67.4	40.2	47.4
Graduate	78.4	76.8	58.5	33.0	67.4	96.9	50.9	39.2	8.8	43.7
Total	56.3	85.7	81.1	51.8	68.4	48.5	63.7	52.1	41.5	54.3

Source: Own calculations from ENOE (II 2019) and ETOE

Additionally, the effect of social distancing on employment will vary significantly depending on the economic sectors: while tourism, the entertainment industry and aviation will be severely affected in the short term, other sectors such as Medical services, food processing and telecommunications will be favoured by the health crisis.

For most of the 15 million Mexicans employed in the informal sector (ENOE, the fourth quarter of 2019), staying home to follow the indications of social distancing that the government has recommended means ceasing to generate the income that allows them to survive every day. Many have to choose between exposing themselves to the virus or starving. It is very likely that the population in this sector will be much more exposed to the effects of the virus, in addition to suffering a drop in their income due to the economic crisis generated by the distancing. The effects of the crisis will be disproportionately high in this sector of the economy.

The return of Mexicans from the United States, who will be affected by the unemployment generated in that country, is another challenge posed by the pandemic to the Mexican labour market. As happened in the 2008-2009 crisis, immigrants have been the hardest hit early on by the COVID19 crisis, because of their relative youth and lower levels of formal education. However, the main reason for the disproportionate increase in migrant unemployment is their concentration in service industries such as retail trade and leisure and hospitality. It has also been shown that, unlike the previous recession, the current economic freefall is affecting women much more than men. The group most affected—Latina immigrants—has the highest unemployment rate of any group, at 22 per cent (Capps, Batalova, & Gelatt, 2020).

In some migrant-expelling localities, the return of population not only puts pressure on the local labour market, but also represents an epidemiological challenge due to exposure to contagion, in places with few medical services.

To this, we must add that the flow of remittances may diminish because of the return of migrants and income reduction of those who remain in the United States. However, contrary to this type of expectations, remittances from the United States to Mexico recorded a record figure ($4,007 million) in March 2020, implying a growth of 35.8% compared to the same month of the previous year. In April the amount went back to $2,861 million still above the amount registered in February. It should be noted that this unusual growth in remittances in March was not observed in other countries with major diasporas in the United States, such as Guatemala and El Salvador. One of the main drivers of the surge in remittances is the 25% increase in the exchange rate of the Mexican peso relative to the dollar. In the face of the depreciation of the peso (instead of devaluation of the peso), Mexicans in the U.S. decided to raise their shipments because the value of remittances increased significantly in real terms and the impact on familiar well-being is much greater. Increased remittances may also indicate a decision to return to Mexico in the medium term in light of the grim future for migrants in the United States.

The loss of employment in Mexico may also lead to the fact that, despite the pandemic has exacerbated xenophobic reactions in the United States and that it is well known that border control has tightened, many Mexicans might start seeing migration to the United States as the only way to get an income for their family. This may have the effect of promoting irregular migration to the North.

Finally, the effects of the pandemic on the already very weak Central American economies will also generate very strong pressures on their labour markets and therefore on migration. It is highly probable that migratory flows to Mexico will grow, and it will be a challenge for our country to manage them without undermining the human rights of migrants and controlling the spread of the pandemic, in an environment that fosters the intensification of anti-immigrant reactions.

The pandemic teaches us that there are no limits to its spread and that the well-being of one sector of the population depends on that of the others. The most prepared to face the pandemic effects seem to be those with the highest levels of human capital, and those inserted in the formal sector. Despite the increase in the schooling levels in Mexico, it is highly likely that the poor quality of education is placing even workers with a University title in a vulnerable situation. Among them, men seem to be more sensitive to the changes that the pandemic is causing in the Mexican labour market. Today, more than ever, it is necessary to implement strategies that, avoiding stigmatizing the most vulnerable population, help them maintain a minimum level of well-being through a well-designed economic and social policy that may include, among other measures, unconditional transfers to those most in need.

References

Campos, R., Esquivel, G., & Lustig, N. (2014). The rise and fall of income inequality in Mexico, 1989-2010. In G. A. Comia, Falling Inequality in Latin America: Policy changes and lessons. Oxford: UNU-WIDER Studies in Development Economics.

Capps, R., Batalova, J., & Gelatt, J. (2020). COVID-19 and Unemployment Assessing the Early Fallout for Immigrants and Other U.S. Workers. Washington, DC: Migration Policy Institute, Fact Sheet.

INEGI. (2020). Resultados de la encuesta telefónica de ocupación y empleo (etoe) cifras oportunas de abril de 2020. Mexico: INEGI.

Kihato, C. W., & Landau, L. (2020). Coercion or the social contract? COVID 19 and spatial (in)justice in African cities. City and Society.

Levy, S. (2018). Esfuerzos mal recompensados: la elusiva búsqueda de la prosperidad en México. Washington, D.C: Banco Interamericano de Desarrollo (Interamerican Development Bank).

Levy, S., & Lopez-Calva, L. F. (2016). Labor Earnings, misallocation , and the returns to education in Mexico. Washingon, D.C.: IDB Working Paper Series, No. IDB-WP-671, Inter-American Development Bank (IDB).

Meza, L., & Rodriguez, R. (In process). Technological change and the Mexican labor market revisited. . Estudios Económicos.

CHAPTER 9

REFLECTIONS ON COLLECTIVE INSECURITY AND VIRTUAL RESISTANCE IN THE TIME OF COVID-19 IN MALAYSIA

Linda Alfarero Lumayag, Teresita C. Del Rosario and Frances S. Sutton

Introduction

No one escapes insecurity today. It is one of the most basic human experiences, more pronounced in others depending on their personal and social circumstances. Personal insecurities refer to the subjective feeling of anxiety and to the concrete lack of protection. This paper attempts to interrogate collective insecurity particularly among migrant workers. The paper likewise argues that such experience gives rise to a form of collective resistance which has become more pronounced within the context of the coronavirus pandemic. In this paper, we argue that migrant insecurity is a collective experience, and is all the more heightened in the context of the coronavirus pandemic. (see for example, Cohen, 2020). We further argue that forms of resistance have been developed as a response to collective insecurity.

Previous studies on insecurity derive mainly from earlier security studies that focused on a broader conceptualisation of nation-states, sovereignty, territoriality and nationalism following the principle of Westphalianism (Vietti & Scribner, 2013). In security studies, migration is framed at the level of institutions, organisations and nation-states and thus, 'securitisation' bias becomes dominant. Migration is a security problem according to this framework, and thus a problem that needs to be addressed through institutional and organisational responses from the state.

This paper looks at insecurity from a micro-level but it also connects these micro-level subjectivities to the macro-realities of state power and its apparatuses. This investigation provides insights into the minute, taken-for-granted ruptures, tensions, fears, conflicts and uncertainties as migrant workers attempt to negotiate the power of the state and its apparatus. In times of crisis, these negotiations become more acute as migrants respond to different forms of insecurity occasioned by the pandemic. These forms include the prospects of hunger, unemployment, and the potential for arrest and deportation. This paper further inquires into possible forms for activities and whether these are sustainable within the context of challenging social, religious, and political milieus in Malaysia.

Malaysia is a particularly interesting case for investigation of migrant insecurity because of the country's response to the demand for global migrant labour. Entrants of labour migrants into the country via legal and illegal channels have been ongoing for the past several decades. It has become a hub for migration in Asia, and the country, unlike other Asian countries, is both a labour-sending and labour-receiving country. Filipinos and Indonesians constitute a major segment for in-migration, whereas Malaysians themselves are migrant labourers in neighbouring Singapore.

A major factor that produces migrant insecurity is the lack of a comprehensive migration policy. Malaysia has yet to address various allegations of migrant insecurities related to work conditions among migrations, social protection and migrant welfare measures (Piper and Rother, 2011; Lee 2018) not to mention civil and political rights.

Observations of this study are based on an ongoing research and our engagement with migrant workers from Indonesia and the Philippines, with a focus on workers in the domestic and service industries. These observations have been the staple of our research and writing for several years prior to the COVID outbreak.

Framing Collective Insecurity

Cohen (2020: 406) proposes that, "insecurities spring from fear, dread of loss, anxiety and uncertainty." Migrant workers experience these insecurities within their own households even before they decide to embark on a migration journey (Cohen and Sirkeci, 2011). Their experiences with poverty, joblessness, lack of opportunities for upward mobility are but a few of their personal circumstances that urge them to contemplate labour migration as a strategy to overcome these various forms of what Del Rosario and Rigg (2019) refer to as "conditions of precarity." Further, Cohen states that "insecurity is a way to represent the collapse of security through time and in response to the assumption of security that may (or may not) have existed, but that nevertheless become concrete and real through history." The two-pronged understanding of insecurity We.e. a psychological/subjective emotion and the absence of adequate protection through policy measures through state interventions guides the analysis of this paper. Subjective security, where it exists, does not necessarily mean that there are protective policies to generate a feeling of security, as institutional and contextual factors (see for example, Chung & Mau, 2014) play an important role to achieve security. Hacker (2006: 20) further argues that, "insecurity requires real risk that threatens real hardship." In a situation of economic insecurity, as demonstrated by the COVID-19 pandemic, joblessness, job displacement and unemployment provide illustrations of a difficult situation from which to draw comparisons between past experiences and practices. Presumably, security has a large psychological component that is linked to feelings of anxiety and safety, which is heavily dependent on personal encounters and circumstances. Economic insecurity, according to the United Nations Department of Economic and Social Affairs (2008: vi), arises from the "exposure of individuals, communities and countries to adverse events, and from their inability to cope with and recover from the costly consequences of those events."

Collective Insecurity Among Migrant workers

In Southeast Asia, Malaysia, Singapore and Thailand are the destination countries of labour migrants from neighbouring countries throughout the region. Malaysia and Thailand are particularly unique in that they are both labour-sending and labour-receiving countries. From a mere half a million at the turn of the millennium, today there are about 5-6 million migrant workers employed across industries, primarily in the construction and manufacturing sectors. Malaysia is a destination country but it also sends workers to Singapore, Hong Kong, Japan and China in a different work package that still remains invisible, unregulated and negligible. Malaysia has been a country entirely reliant on the presence of immigrants/migrant workers before and after colonial rule (Kassim, 2013; Kaur 2014; Lumayag, 2018). Plantation industry relies on labour migrants from southern India during the British times to Indonesia and Bangladesh under present administration.

Migrant insecurity in Malaysia is best described in the context of a sustained and prolonged feeling of job insecurity that is reflected in the daily interactions of migrants and the State. Piper et al. (2016: 1096)) succinctly notes that,

Foreign employment demands to be understood as precarious work under taken to mitigate existing conditions of precarity at home, generally structured by historical and ongoing processes of uneven development. The fundamental problem is not only the insecurity and vulnerability associated with migrant labour, but the lack of opportunities, rights, security and protection at home that causes large segments of the labour force to resort to migration as a survival strategy or in pursuit of aspirations for social upward mobility.

Insecurities among migrants became more pronounced during partial lockdown, known as MCO (Movement Control Order), for almost three months. These we term 'modalities' which have been around for years, and remain contentious issues for migrants, civil society movements and governments of sending and receiving countries. These modalities pre-exist embedding psychological, subjective experiences of migrant labour conditions across different sectors of the Malaysian economy. However, when COVID-19 was first detected in Malaysia, a new modality came into practice.

Modalities of insecurities are as follows: employment conditions (Lumayag, 2018, 2020a, 2020b; Kassim, 2013); restriction against formation of labour union (Piper, 2013, 2015; Piper et al., 2016); lack of social protection mechanisms (Piper and Uhlin, 2002); access/(or lack of) to legal redress (Piper and Uhlin, 2002; Sadiq, 2005); racism, moral panic and xenophobia (Sadiq, 2005; Lyons, 2007); weak governance on bribery and corruption; and, weak worker protection from labour sending governments. The tendency to leave migrant's rights unaddressed by global and national institutions is the result of institutional failures at all levels, lack of political will to respond to the human costs involved in temporary contract migration (Chi, 2008, as cited in Piper et al., 2016), and the downward spiral with regard to labour standards globally (Munck, 2002, as cited in Piper et al., 2016).

After the Perikatan Nasional (PN) government took over the national leadership (23 February 2020), the MCO was declared and implemented. The unprecedented crisis has put Malaysia in a standstill. Not only did it affect the citizens but it affected the non-Malaysians even more. About 12000 attendees of an Islamic religious movement called the Tabligh,1 including about 2000 Rohingya refugees gathered in a Sri Petaling mosque, Kuala Lumpur on 27 February - 1 March. This cluster was partly responsible for the spike in the number of COVID-19 cases in West Malaysia, Sabah and Sarawak. The Malaysian government found it challenging to do contact tracing especially for the undocumented Tabligh members. In fact, some narratives that demonstrate resistance to subject members to health testing was as divine reckoning. As of 24 May, 115 deaths were recorded with over 7000 cases of infection, about 50% of which came from the Sri Petaling cluster. Other clusters were reportedly linked to the Emmanuel Baptist Church in Sarawak, a political party dinner and a St. Joseph's Day gathering, in Kuching.

Virtual resistance as a form of activism: MCO and COVID-19

While investigations in the past revolved around open confrontations against power (Foucault, ; Constable, 1997; Parreñas, 2001), the current crisis provides opportunities for new ways of understanding the minute, invisible political actions of vulnerable groups. Seminal studies demonstrate the

---

[1] Tabligh is a religious movement with vast numbers of followers from all over Asia, which makes it a major social force underpinned by religious belief.

variety of actions of resistance among vulnerable groups (Scott 1985, 1990; Ong, 1987; Constable 1997; Chin 1998; and Lumayag 2018). Scott's focus is on everyday resistance among peasants in rural Malaysia, where Constable, Chin and Lumayag illustrate the outright use of state power in reducing opportunities for marginalised groups to confront the state. In all these studies, the resistance of marginalised, vulnerable minorities are conducted in the open, hastened by physical, spatial and social 'presence' such as when they confront their powerful employers. In these settings, migrant resistance is a community-based form of active engagement that is fleeting, and is expressed in micro activities to respond to a threat or threats to one's basic survival. These threats form the basis on why migrant workers feel extremely insecure in at least two domains: the loss of job, and therefore hunger for their families back home, and digital surveillance of the State. These micro activities are often invisible in the public eye, and carried out in ways that unless one belongs to the group, one does not comprehend the full extent of its efficacy.

What is common in these studies is active participation of vulnerable groups through forms of engagement that are conducted individually, away from the prying eyes of the powerful employers or agents. Activism is performed on a different platform with the introduction of the internet in which the sharing of information holds the key to active engagement (see earlier studies by Anderson, 2013 on the Arab Spring; Costa, 2013 on Turkey; Miller et al., 2016). Altogether, the widespread use of the internet becomes collective action, rather than conducted and carried out by individual workers. Because migrant workers can make use of common platforms and share their insecurities, the individual sharing of experiences becomes a motivating factor to extend assistance to each other and help understand their common situations of insecurity. Echoing Scott, online presence becomes another "weapons of the weak" in the current situation where migrants workers are left isolated, discriminated against and rendered vulnerable as COVID-19 continues to infect society.

Migrants are easy targets because of how they are viewed and regarded in society. Bauman (2016) reveals that in Europe, for example, the 'migration crisis' has triggered a deluge of racism and xenophobia, thus creating divisions of "insiders/outsiders", "us/them", and "all the others." As explained earlier in Hall's (1978) 'moral panic' phenomenon and Michael Bakhtin's concept of 'cosmic fear', (in Bauman 1998), migrants take away job opportunities intended for citizens, the "insiders", and the "rightful" recipients of rights. In similar vein, Foucault's (1997) notion of "biopolitics" raise the same issues as Bakhtin and Bauman. On the one hand, foreign workers are viewed as "dirty", yet society allows them to work in the homes and take good care of citizens, serve in restaurants, eating stalls or big malls where cleanliness and hygiene are requirements for maintenance and continuity of these various places.

As a response, migrant workers attempt to defy notions of 'racialised' bodies by creating enclaves of migrant communities in society (Lyons, 2007). The effective domination of power speaks of worker's embodiment of roles and position that would have great repercussion on one's economic position, or flexible citizenship (Ong, 1999) in a transnational social space. Nonetheless, as Foucault (1997) would have impressed, power is relational, that it also resides in the realm of the powerless. This also suggests affinity with Scott's (1985, 1990) classic material on the 'weapons of the weak' for the subordinate, oppressed and socially excluded group of people, the migrant workers.

When the MCO was declared, the PN government opened a massive relief package ('care' package) of RM250 billion (approx. US$58 m) to cushion the negative economic impact of COVID-19 on the citizens of the country. The relief package was extended to the lowest economic category of B40[2] up to the employers of small and business enterprises. Interestingly, the non-citizens, specifically the documented and undocumented immigrants and migrants and refugees, were not included in the 'care' package. As the MCO progressed, calls of food aid come from migrant workers, the daily waged workers, who were stuck in their flats when employers refused to provide them food to sustain them during the days when they were without work.

Two local-based migrant NGOs, namely, Our Journey and AMMPO-*Asosasyon ng mga Manggagawang Pilipino Overseas Malaysia*[3], started organising the distribution of food aid packages4 to live-out Filipino and Indonesian domestic workers around Kuala Lumpur, Petaling Jaya and immediate environs. Everyday both leading groups received requests that ranged from food to diapers, formula milk and sanitary pads. The Our Journey teams purchased and distributed relief packages; meanwhile, AMMPO screened through the aid list, with names, locations and mobile numbers of affected migrant workers. As the food aid continued, Our Journey negotiated and collaborated with foreign embassies such as the Indonesian and Bangladeshi embassies to reach out to affected thousands of migrant workers. Migrant workers sought food assistance when their employers abandoned them without paying their wages and absconded with their passports. Apart from domestic work, work in the service and construction industries were seriously affected. Those who worked in restaurants, hotels, hawker stalls, massage

---

[2] B40 is a category of household whose mean income is RM2,537 and a median income of RM2,629.
[3] Association of Filipino Workers Overseas.
[4] Food aid packages contained 5 kg of rice, 1 liter cooking oil, 5 cans sardines, 1 kg sugar, 1 pack of 3-in-1 coffee, 1 kg noodles, 5 packs instant noodles, 1 tray (30 pcs) eggs, onions and garlic.

parlours or in the construction industry - masonry and welding – found themselves stranded. Since movement was restricted and implementation was very strict, the team needs to show a permit issued by a foreign embassy to allow distribution to their nationals when passing a police roadblock. Earlier, NGOs were required to send all donations to the government for distribution through the Ministry of Welfare but later the restriction was withdrawn due to widespread protests from NGOs. Also, the NGOs wanted to demonstrate the performance of goodwill towards the migrant community in as much as they are receiving donations for this purpose.

During the MCO, the Federal leadership pledged that a moratorium on arrests and detention for millions of undocumented workers would take effect. However, this was not the case. On 01 May, organised arrests and detention occurred in downtown Kuala Lumpur along with Jalan Masjid India where Malaya Mansion and Selangor Mansion are located, the cluster that was thought to have started the spike of coronavirus infection among the migrant workers. More than 500 undocumented workers were rounded up in a raid and sent to the nearest immigration depot and were promised a mass testing thereafter. Although they tested negative of the virus, the fact that their immigration status is undocumented, the government reneged on its earlier promise not to arrest them. This discriminatory action against the migrant communities triggered online protests coordinated by several labour unions, migrant communities and NGOs. The United Nations office in Kuala Lumpur also condemned the arrests and instead offered to find alternatives to detention in a press statement shared widely. The global network of migration groups engaged in advocacy and human rights issues organised webinar discussions and suggested potential strategies should the spate of arrests continue during the MCO. Even the plan to centralise the distribution of food aid to citizens and non-citizens was vehemently resisted by local groups and civil society organisations. Away from the listening ear of State actors, the public message was to control and dominate the relief operations, in addition to a persistent feeling that the State wanted to monitor the locations of undocumented workers. When the Philippine Embassy urged the distribution teams of Our Journey and AMMPO to provide them with the list before the Embassy can release its letter of consent to allow the food distribution to Filipino nationals, both groups reacted strongly against this demand. The undocumented workers preferred to rely on migrant groups viz-a-viz the Embassy that represented the sending country (e.g., Philippines, Indonesia, Bangladesh). The process of documenting the distribution was to preserve anonymity, thanks to masks that recipients are obliged to wear outside the house premises.

In Sarawak, undocumented workers in the massage and beauty salons, restaurants and construction sector, almost numbering one hundred in the second week of the MCO, found it extremely difficult to survive since there was work stoppage. Employers temporarily abandoned their workers and some thought they were already retrenched without the workers knowing their work status. Sarawak holds a relatively high number of undocumented foreign workers, estimated at around 300,000 in 2015.[5]

The case of abuse of state power is demonstrated in the following incident. During the third week of the MCO, two community leaders received persistent calls allegedly from someone representing state authorities inquiring whether the particular Embassy is sending money to purchase food packs for its nationals working in Sarawak, and if the community leaders wanted their (callers) his assistance to do the food deliveries. Initially the plan was to distribute the deliveries on their own by visiting them at home. The call from the alleged friendly officers revised the plan for food distribution. Instead of the traditional way of handing the goods to recipients, have a photo taken, and perhaps upload them on Facebook for documentation and public sharing, that strategy is no longer possible. Like in Kuala Lumpur, where there is strict adherence to movement protocols, one chilling measure is for uniform personnel to accompany the distribution team to each and every location of beneficiaries thereby putting the security of all undocumented at risk. So the call from the 'friendly' officer hastened to shift the strategy by going low profile. The community leaders were quick to shift the strategy by negotiating with local grocers to deliver the food pack directly to undocumented workers without a trace of any physical movement. It was also not a necessity to take photos and share on Facebook, unlike what Kuala Lumpur teams had done. And because FB accounts of recipients are suddenly decorated of food rations, the rumour mill went on overdrive that most photo uploads of food recipients suddenly disappeared in less than a few hours. Most online surveys also stopped and there was advisory not to entertain any online surveys especially for the undocumented until they know where the online survey originated.

In one area, authorities wondered why migrant workers were silent and with that, the community leaders were informed again that this 'friendly officer' received a call from the Embassy informing him of plan to distribute food packs after the MCO. Also, authorities must be informed and if aid is sent to the area, he should be made aware of it.

Undocumented Indonesian workers in the construction industry relied mostly on their local friends to survive. One positive action done by the Embassy of Indonesia was to facilitate the smooth distribution of food aid packages across geographical locations from Kuala Lumpur to Shah Alam,

---

[5] https://www.malaymail.com/news/malaysia/2015/04/11/illegal-immigrants-in-sarawak-a-huge-problem-deputy-home-minister-admits/876739.

Klang and in the Selangor areas and across states in West Malaysia. The Indonesian Embassy may have realised that it was impossible to reach out to migrant workers without logistical assistance from civil society groups and migrant communities. One Indonesian group of domestic workers (PERTIMIG6- Persatuan Pekerja Rumah Tangga Indonesia Migran) in Kuala Lumpur with an alliance with a labour union in Hong Kong organised the list of recipients and followed the distribution by keeping the private and organisation donors of food aid informed. Indonesian workers have a higher representation of undocumented workers because of the shared and porous borders between Indonesia and East Malaysia and the Peninsula.

Since non-citizens do not receive any form of assistance from the PN government, migrant workers rely on assistance by establishing new networks, link up with other Kuala Lumpur-based associations and migrant communities and extend as much help as they can even if it means to receive less in the process. For instance, their domestic worker friends who live with employers quietly send rations to other friends across geographical locations without leaving their employers' homes. Their established Grab or taxi contacts are employed to ferry these rations to friends who live out of their employers' homes. At times, those live-out friends collect the goods from live-in domestic workers, then prepare or cook them and pack for those in need. For example, baking bread by ten pieces and then distributed to friends. It is safe to say that migrant workers in Malaysia survived the MCO mainly from assistance from well-meaning Malaysian private individuals. In some cases, employers of live-in foreign domestic workers attempted to "adopt" a few migrant workers and their families, provided them with basic foodstuffs to survive through the movement restriction. Nonetheless, there are complaints from employees whose employers who did not provide food for their workers. A story of J (name withheld), 32 years old, undocumented, worked in a restaurant for 11 months before the MCO. J reasoned that husband-wife owners of the restaurant were good. Although, since the beginning of the MCO, his employers never asked him whether he had food to eat. He was also not paid since the partial lockdown. We then asked J if he still thought if his employers were good, to which he just kept silent. According to J, he did not want to sound too demanding by asking, because he was afraid that after the MCO he would be asked to leave the workplace like what he has been hearing from friends. J wanted to earn to buy a plane ticket and to pay the compound fee for overstaying which he did not know the cost. Another group of five wood furniture makers experienced hunger amidst plenty of stocks of rice and piles of noodles in the warehouse owned by their employer. The employer never offered anything since the MCO began. When a local religious charity arm offered them food and RM200

---

6 PERTIMIG is Association of Indonesian Migrant Domestic Workers.

(approx. US$46) cash per worker, they were overcome by emotion.

Most migrant workers have Facebook accounts, but during the MCO, the undocumented workers' accounts were not actively online, preferring instead to lie low, but the WhatsApp account was more lively. Some Indonesian workers use their documented friends' names to link to NGOs like Our Journey, AMMPO and PERTIMIG to escape surveillance.

Although Malaysian citizens may have received cash assistance from the Federal and State governments, a number of undocumented internal migrant workers who cannot access the application via the online government system were left out in the process. Instead, these migrants relied on their friendship cliques with foreign workers. Thus, a small number of internal migrants benefitted as well from the generosity of fellow migrants, as observed in East Malaysia.

Other manifestations of migrants' ability to fight off surveillance are to deny that they received any form of assistance to pool food supplies they have collected. One group knew that their request for food assistance would most likely be denied by the Philippine government. Yet, when the list reached a migrant advocacy group in Kuala Lumpur, the group referred the request to the office of the Welfare Attache for the Overseas Welfare Work Association (OWWA) and the request was granted quickly in less than three days. Seventeen families with children received a food pack worth RM40 (approx. US$9) each per family. We did an online chat in one of the recipients and said that "we are just testing the waters, if the government gives well and good, if it doesn't, at least we tried."

Conclusion: forging a new engagement through virtual activism?

Amidst abundant threats today, human insecurity is omnipresent. The onset of COVID-19 globally and the ensuing MCO lockdown in Malaysia brought the economy to its knees. Most affected are the daily waged earners B40 and 85% of migrant workers in the small and medium industries, in addition to foreign domestic workers confined in private homes. Millions of migrant workers are located in non-essential services such as domestic work, beauty salons, hotels and restaurants. At the lifting of the MCO, some workers were already issued an exit pass, while other workers wait it out and reconsider plans of returning home.

Could the new socio-political landscape as a result of pandemic give way to a new mode of engagement that is more virtually visible? While workers are able to wait out the crisis and survived the critical two months under confinement because of engagement with other migrant communities or have forged new alliances with advocacy groups (Hansen, 2019), would they sustain the kind of virtual political engagement to mitigate insecurities and to improve their work conditions (Gurowitz, 2000; Basok, 2010; Piper et al., 2016)? Will this crisis lay the groundwork to push for more social protection? At the same time, would the pandemic engender a deepened digital surveillance that risks civil liberties and rights, just as when migrant workers realised the importance of virtual resistance to achieve change? These questions raise possibilities for generating new knowledge that would help understand the new landscape for human action within the context of a global pandemic.

References

Anderson, C. W. (2013). Youth, the "Arab Spring and Social Movements. Review of Middle East Studies, 47 (2), 150-156

Basok, T. (2010). Opening a dialogue on migrant (rights) activism. Studies in Social Justice, 4(2): 97. Retrieved from https://search.proquest.com/docview/ 1315917773?accountid=40705

Bauman, Z. (1998). In Search of Politics. UK: Polity Press

Bauman, Z. (2016). Strangers at our Door. UK: Polity Press

Chin, C. B. N. (1998). In service and servitude: Foreign female domestic workers and the Malaysian "modernity" project. New York: Columbia University Press.

Chung, H. and S. Mau (2014). Subjective insecurity ad the role of institutions. Journal of European Social Policy, 24(4): 303-318

Cohen, J. H. (2020). Editorial: Modeling Migration, Insecurity and COVID-19. Migration Letters, 17(3): 405-410

Cohen, J. H. and I. Sirkeci (2011). Cultures of migration: the global nature of contemporary mobility. Austin: University of Texas Press

Constable, N. (1997). Maid to order in Hong Kong: Stories of Filipina workers. Ithaca & London: Cornell University Press

Costa, E. (2013). The Wider World: politics, the visible and invisible. *Social Media in Southeast Turkey,* 3(1): 128-162

Del Rosario, T. C. and J. Rigg (2019). Introduction. "Special Issue on Precarity in Asia." *Journal of Contemporary Asia,* 49(4): 517-527. https://www.tandfonline.com/doi/full/10.1080/00472336.2019.1581832

Foucault, M. (1997). Society Must be Defended. New York City, NY, USA: Picador

Gurowitz, A. (2000). Migrant rights and activism in Malaysia: Opportunities and constraints. The Journal of Asian Studies, 59(4): 863-888.

Hacker, J. S. (2006). The Great Risk Shift: The Assault on American Jobs, Families and Health Care, and Retirement and How you can Fight Back. New York: Oxford University Press

Hall, S. (1978). Policing the Crisis: Mugging, the state and law 'n' order. London: Macmillan

Hansen, C. (2019). Solidarity in Diversity: Activism as a Pathway of Migrant Emplacement in Melano. Doctoral Thesis, University of Malmo

The Malay Mail. https://www.malaymail.com/news/malaysia/2015/04/11/illegal-immigrants-in-sarawak-a-huge-problem-deputy-home-minister-admits/876739

Kassim, A. (2013). Current trends in transnational population in Malaysia: Issues, policy and challenges. In: International Population Conference on Migration, Urbanisation & Development. Unpublished work, Faculty of Economics and Administration, University of Malaya

Kaur, A. (2014). Managing labour migration in Malaysia: Guest worker programs and the regularisation of irregular labour migrants as a policy instrument. Asian Studies Review, 38(3), 345–366

Lee, J. C. H. (2018). Women's Activism in Malaysia. Voices and Insights. Cham, Switzerland: Palgrave Pivot. https://doi.org/10.1007/978-3-319-78969-9

Lyons, L. (2007). Dignity Overdue: Women's Rights Activism in Support of Foreign Domestic Workers in Singapore. Women's Studies Quarterly 35(3): 106-122.

Lumayag, L.A. (2018). Contesting Disciplinary Power: Transnational Domestic Labour in the Global South. Asian Studies Review, 42(1): 161-177. DOI: 10.1080/10357823.2017.1413072

Lumayag, L. A. (2020a). Undocumented migrants: strangers, 'moral panics' and betrayal of trust. https://aliran.com/thinking-allowed-online/strangers-moral-panics-and-betrayal-of-trust/

Lumayag, L. A. (2020b). Fear, now hunger: undocumented in the time of coronavirus. https://aliran.com/thinking-allowed-online/fear-now-hunger-undocumented-in-the-time-of-coronavirus/ [Accessed: 13/08/2020].

Miller, D. et al. (2016). How the World Changed Social Media. California: UCL Press. http://www.jstor.org/stable/j.ctt1g69z35.9

Ong, A. (1987). Spirits of resistance and capitalist discipline: Factory women in Malaysia. New York: State University of New York Press

Ong, A. (1999). Flexible Citizenship: The Cultural Logics of Transnationality. UK: Duke University Press

Parreñas, R. (2001). Servants of globalisation: Women, migration and domestic work. Stanford: Stanford University Press.

Piper, N. (2013). 'Resisting Inequality: Global Migrant Rights Activism'. In T. Bastia (ed.) Migration and Inequality, pp. 45–64. New York: Routledge

Piper, N. (2015). 'Democratising Migration from the Bottom Up: The Rise of the Global Migrant Rights Movement', Globalizations, 12(5): 788–802

Piper, N. and S. Rother (2011). 'Transnational Inequalities, Transnational Responses: The Politicisation of Migrant Rights in Asia'. In B. Rehbein (ed.) Globalisation and Inequality in Emerging Societies, pp. 235–55. London: Palgrave Macmillan

Piper, N. and A. Uhlin (2002). Transnational advocacy networks and the issue of female labour migration and trafficking in East and South East Asia: A gendered analysis of opportunities and obstacles. Asian and Pacific Migration Journal, 11(2): 171-196

Piper, N. et al. (2016). Redefining a Rights-based approach in the context of temporary labour migration in Asia. UNRISD Working Papers 2016-11. http://www.unrisd.org/80256B3C005BCCF9/(httpAuxPages)/72E2E53E545B067BC12580250043BA1D/$file/Piper%20et%20al.pdf

Sadiq, K. (2005). When states prefer non-citizens over citizens: Conflict over illegal immigration into Malaysia. International Studies Quarterly, 49(1), 101–122

Scott, J. (1985). Weapons of the weak: Everyday forms of peasant resistance. New Haven & London: Yale University Press

Scott, J. (1990). Domination and the arts of resistance – hidden transcripts. New Haven & London: Yale University Press

United Nations Department of Economic and Social Affairs (2008) 'World Economic and Social Survey 2008: Overcoming Economic Insecurity', http://www.un.org/en/development/desa/policy/ wess/wess_archive/2008wess.pdf

Vietti, F. and T. Scribner (2013). Human Insecurity: Understanding International Migration from a Human Security Perspective. Journal on Migration and Human Security, 1: 17-31.

CHAPTER 10

FACING A PANDEMIC AWAY FROM HOME: COVID-19 AND THE BRAZILIAN IMMIGRANTS IN PORTUGAL

Patricia Posch and Rosa Cabecinhas

Introduction

On January 7, 2020, the Portuguese newspaper, *Público,* published an article about an unprecedented challenge facing Chinese leaders: a "strange form of pneumonia" (Chaiça, 2020) diagnosed in several patients in the Chinese city of Wuhan, that was subsequently named COVID-19. On March 2, the Portuguese government had placed major hospitals under alert and reinforced the supply of medicines (Campos & Lins, 2020). This occurred even before the declaration of a global pandemic by the World Health Organisation, on March 12 (WHO, 2020), and diagnosis of the first cases in Portugal. On March 18, a national state of emergency was declared - which imposed social measures, such as social isolation and mobility restrictions in public spaces. The state of emergency continued until May 2, when it was replaced by the state of calamity, and then by the state of contingency on July 1.

Covid-19 has another ironic or perverse trait. It does not reach everyone in the same way. It may even be a seductive speech that we are in the same boat, but it's not real (Severo, 2020, Chapter 24, para. 7).

While such challenges were affecting Portuguese society, immigrants began to face a different set of concerns, that placed their lives in even more vulnerable situations. Along with refugees and racialised persons – who, despite being national citizens, are perceived as foreigners - various groups of immigrants are seen as the "Other" and stigmatised because they are viewed as a threat in the destination country. As stated by Paéz and Pérez (2020), in an epidemic scenario, the hegemonic collective often 'foreignises' the disease – i.e. associates it with outgroup individuals. This stigmatisation is something that Vala and Pereira (2020) relate to the worldwide reinforcement of national identities, anti-universalistic beliefs and the rise of political governments aligned with right-wing values. Although it can be claimed that this is used by dominant social groups to reduce anxiety and increase their sense of control over the situation, fostering a false impression that they are less vulnerable to the disease (Smith, O'Connor & Joffe, 2015), one should not forget that, within social processes[1], scapegoating is one of the most extreme forms of prejudice against groups that are socially blamed for causing another group's misfortunes (Glick, 2005).

Indeed, in times of public health disturbances, history shows that such processes of social segregation based on scapegoating are not rare. For example, the unprecedented 1889–1890 flu pandemic was called the 'Asiatic flu' or 'Russian flu'. The most evident case is the 1918 influenza pandemic. The sole fact that the disease was called the 'Spanish flu' even though it did not originate in Spain (Hoppe, 2018) corroborates the idea that "Others" are frequently identified as being the causes of such diseases. This is particularly true for individuals who belong to social groups that are perceived as having low social status. In Portugal, Galician immigrants were stigmatised throughout the three waves of the Spanish influenza, which reflected the waves occurring worldwide, although we now know that the first wave of the spread of the disease began in the Alentejo region, in the rural area of Portugal. In the second wave, it spread from the city of Porto to the Northwest and Douro region, followed by the Centre and finally, the South of Portugal (Sobral & Lima, 2018).

Bearing this in mind, while it can be assumed that a pandemic often brings a sense of unity to social groups that share a fear of the potential impact of a virus on all human beings, regardless of their social positioning, it also highlights the disparities of social positions and the dilemmas that different social groups face in a given society. The same finding applies to Brazilian immigrants in Portugal, the largest community of documented foreign residents living in Portugal. In 2019, according to official statistics, there were 151,304 documented Brazilian immigrants in Portugal, equivalent to 25.6% of all documented immigrants living in the country (SEF, 2020). This reflects the historical migratory flow from Brazil to Portugal, that became more firmly consolidated in the 1980s. The main driver of this trend was the fact that as the Brazilian economy entered a period of an unprecedented deceleration, Portugal has begun to emerge as an alternative for those seeking better opportunities and quality of life, mainly due to the fact that the country joined the European Economic Community (EEC) in 1986. This migratory flow began as a countercurrent movement, since many Brazilians immigrants were part of the family of former Portuguese emigrants returning to their homeland. But it was soon complemented by the emigration of highly qualified professionals and political exiles. In the mid-1990s, Portugal joined

---

[1] Scapegoating processes can be understood as a social practice, in alignment with socially-shared beliefs, ideologies and stereotypes embedded in a given cultural context (Allport, 1954; Glick, 2005).

the Schengen Area[2] and a services-based economy began to emerge, which attracted Brazilians with a more diversified profile. In this second migratory wave, Brazilian immigrants with lower educational levels began to occupy the least qualified positions in the Portuguese job market, in particular in the food and tourism sectors (Padilla, Marques, Góis & Peixoto, 2015). The feminisation observed in migratory movements in other parts of the world can also be observed here. Although the statistics showed only a 2% difference between the number of Brazilian women and men living in Portugal in 2003, this difference increased annually[3] and stood at 8% in 2008 (Barbosa & Lima, 2020).

This configuration of the migratory flow continued until the end of the first decade of the new millennium, when it began to show signs of weakening, especially because of the 2008 global economic recession. From 2011 onwards, the number of documented Brazilian immigrants living in Portugal began to fall, which Machado (2014) attributes to return migration or new migration to other European countries. This trend only changed in 2017, when the decline in the number of documented Brazilian immigrants resident in Portugal was replaced by an accelerated upward trend, with a 23.4% increase in 2018 and an even more impressive increase, of 43.5%, in 2019 (SEF, 2020). Not only these numbers, but also the different media discourses that are emerging in relation to the new Brazilian immigrants in Portugal, attest to the existence of a third migratory wave over recent years.

In the context of the COVID-19 pandemic, Brazilian immigrants soon emerged in media discourses, both in Brazil and Portugal, that aimed to explore how they are dealing with a pandemic in a foreign country. Such narratives proliferated and soon began to be generalised - from unemployment to days spent at the airport with no resources and waiting for a flight to return to Brazil. However, although the media now constitutes an important source of information and knowledge (Talbot, 2007), when possible, its supposed factual authority should be questioned and analysed using more in-depth analysis of the underlying topic. Given the size of the Brazilian community resident in Portugal – and hence the important role played by these individuals in Portuguese social and economic structures - we considered that it would be extremely valuable to understand how such individuals have been coping with the COVID-19 pandemic.

---

[2] The Schengen Area represents the geographical area of 26 countries that joined the Schengen Agreement, established in 1985, where there are no border controls of residents from any of the signatory countries, in order to allow free movement of people between countries. (Carvalhais, 2008)

[3] With the exception of 2006, when the number of women decreased by 3%. Nonetheless, they still represented a majority, since women were 51% and men 49% of all documented Brazilian immigrants living in Portugal that year (SEF, 2010).

Methodology

The main goal of this qualitative empirical research is to explore and bring to light the impacts of the COVID-19 pandemic on the lives of Brazilian immigrants in Portugal. With this goal in mind, we developed a script with four major thematic blocks of topics to be used in semi-structured interviews: biographical information, migration trajectory, life in Portugal and perceived impacts of the COVID-19 pandemic.

Acknowledging that this research was not intended to be representative, the respondents were selected using the approach of convenience and opportunity (Tracy, 2020). The sole criterion for the selection of respondents was the year of migration, since the intention was to portray the point of view of Brazilian immigrants from the current third wave (França & Padilla, 2018). A public call was posted in online groups of Brazilians living in Portugal, on *Facebook*, *WhatsApp* and *Telegram*. The interviews were conducted via audio calls made over the Internet, between May 18 and June 22.

In total, 19 people were interviewed, a number that is compatible with that which Gaskell (2003) considers to be ideal for exploring a research topic without undermining the researchers' analytic capacity. 13 of the respondents were women and six were men. The age range was between 23 and 58 years old. Only three of the respondents were single. The others stated that they are married or live in a "stable union" (de facto marriage) with a Brazilian partner. In terms of their educational level, 16 respondents had completed at least a Higher Education degree, and three are currently enrolled in postgraduation courses. In terms of professional status, one respondent was retired, nine worked for companies in Portugal and two were entrepreneurs. The other seven respondents said that they were unemployed, dating back to before the COVID-19 pandemic. In terms of the region where the respondents lived in Brazil prior to migrating to Portugal, 12 lived in the Southeast – Rio de Janeiro, São Paulo, Espírito Santo and Minas Gerais, three in the Northeast – Bahia, Ceará and Pernambuco, three in the South – Paraná and Santa Catarina - and one in the Midwest – Distrito Federal. In Portugal, nine live in the South – Évora, Faro, Lisbon and Setúbal, eight in the North – Aveiro, Porto and Viana do Castelo - and two in the Centre region – Castelo Branco and Coimbra. In relation to the year of migration, nine respondents migrated in 2019 and three in 2020. The other seven respondents migrated between 2015 and 2018.

Although this paper does not aim to provide in-depth analysis of the characteristics of the sample, it is interesting to observe how it can be related to previous migratory waves from Brazil to Portugal and what it tells about the current wave. The fact that more than a half of the respondents were women, for example, can be associated with the tendency of the feminisation of this flow, observed since the second wave. The higher educational level also matches the tendency of higher qualified migrants, that can be attested when comparing this data with that of all migrants from that same flow (Padilla et al., 2015). When it comes to where they lived prior to migration, except for one respondent who lived in Distrito Federal, 12 respondents came from states that were the source of over 50% of the immigrants from the second flow (Padilla et al., 2015), while the other six respondents came from states in the Northeast and South regions, whose representativeness has increased over recent years (Barbosa & Lima, 2020).

Results

First of all, we sought to understand the impact of the pandemic on the lives of the respondents. The backdrop of economic recession - it is impossible to ignore the economic "tumble" that could lead Portugal's GDP to shrink by 6.8% in 2020, which is nonetheless more optimistic than the 7.7% drop in GDP that is forecast for other European Union countries (Francisco, 2020) - ended up having a direct influence on the lives of Brazilian immigrants. For the entrepreneurs in the sample, the pandemic has multiple impacts. Carlos[4] (30), who abandoned his career in Human Resources in Brazil to set up his own business in the food sector in Portugal, admitted that the pandemic had had an impact on his planned business. "Initially, it will open as a take-away and then we will determine how to manage the issue of the virus itself", he stated. Karine (51), who worked in the Marketing sector in Brazil and is now an entrepreneur in the tourism sector in Portugal, considers that the impact of the pandemic makes it necessary to reassess where she should direct the business. "We had a lot, a lot of work, and now we are walking on eggshells", she explained, assuming that, with the pandemic, "a little bit more care" will be needed in all aspects of her company's business. For those who are presently employed, the fear of possible dismissal was reported as being always imminent, despite the fact that the unemployment rate in the first quarter of 2020 in Portugal remained the same as that in the last quarter of 2019 (INE, 2020). This was also portrayed by the media, such as news items which stated that the new coronavirus is "the virus that has brought unemployment to [the Brazilian immigrants]" (Filho, 2020). This concern was referred to by Pedro, who told us that he thinks he has nothing that differentiates him from the other employees of the company where he works, beyond his job performance. "If, for example, the company downsizes and has to fire someone, I'll probably be on the front line," he said, "I'm going to have to be better than anyone else, or they'll dismiss me first". This concern, however, seemed to be less pronounced for those immigrants who, either because of their professional

---

[4] We used fictitious names to protect the anonymity of the respondents.

position or because they are in a different social position, do not feel that their work is threatened by the pandemic. Working in the legal field at a company that provides legal services to Brazil, Liana (27), who migrated to Portugal in 2017 and now works for a law firm, recognises that she is in a different position from those immigrants who are most affected by the pandemic. "I am aware that I am in a privileged position with respect to many immigrants," she said. "Since we audit the Brazilian market, even in the situation of collective dismissal, I even have a little greater job security". There were even immigrants for whom the pandemic offered new opportunities. Juliana (30), who works at an air filter company in Portugal after migrating in 2019, said that sales have increased significantly as a result of the pandemic. "My husband has therefore joined the company, otherwise he would be unemployed now".

Some respondents also revealed that they recognised the impacts of the pandemic on their mental health. "When the world says that an avalanche of mental problems will come, it is no joke", said Karine, for whom the imposition of having to stay at home has been challenging in psychological terms. "I love working from my home-office, but as a result of being forced to stay [inside the house]… I started to freak out", she explained. For Carla (32), who migrated to Portugal in 2017 and now lives in Castelo Branco, surviving the new coronavirus also involves taking care with her mental health, especially because, in her words, "we get a little crazy, feel a little bit alone". This is not an unreasonable concern. Ornell et al. (2020) remind us that, in pandemic scenarios, concern about the pathogen and the biological aspect of the virus ends up overshadowing - or even neglecting - the associated psychological and psychiatric consequences for human beings. According to these authors, fear "increases the levels of anxiety and stress in healthy individuals and intensifies the symptoms of those pre-existing psychiatric disorders" (Ornell, Schuch, Sordi & Kessler, 2020, p. 2). In the case of immigrants, there is still a need to look at, and take care of, mental health as an issue crossing the past and the present, i.e. recognising the influence of individuals' history and migratory trajectory on their mental constitution (Lechner, 2007).

In the case studied, the emergence of situations of social discrimination - one of the most pressing issues facing immigrants - was also reported. In an official statement, issued on March 30, the UN representative, Fernand de Varennes, warned that COVID-19 is not only a health issue, but also a potential agent of exacerbating situations of xenophobia, hatred and social exclusion (Varennes, 2020). This theme also emerged in our research in the account of Carla, who told us that she suffered xenophobia in her workplace because she is Brazilian. "Sometimes, in meetings, I have to listen to 'oh, the Brazilian is here, she will give us COVID-19'," she said. "It is a shame to see the sad plight of Brazilian people becoming a joke at a meeting of a company, that I previously considered to be serious", she added. This "sad plight" is associated to the high incidence of cases of COVID-19 in her native country, which, throughout the month of May, became an epicentre of the pandemic in Latin America and the world (Waldron, 2020). According to Worldometer - a website that compiles world statistics on the new coronavirus - in a consultation carried out at 07:40 GMT on September 1st, the country already ranked second, with 3,910,901 cases, in the global list of countries with the highest number of total registered cases – 25,644,319. While it has already been found that residents in areas of high incidence are more vulnerable to episodes of social discrimination (Ornell et al., 2020), our study reveals that, even when they are no longer residing in the country in question, nationality turns out to be an unavoidable part of immigrants' identity, which leads them to be a target of such disturbances.

On the other hand, the enforcement of social distancing and quarantine affected these immigrants, by restricting their mobility in public spaces, including their routines – "I spent virtually 30 days without even going to the supermarket," said Ana (40), a mother who has been living in Loulé, alone with her young child, since 2019 - and also affected their leisure options - for Juliana, going out to eat; for Pedro, going to the beach. This presence in public spaces, which was also a moment of social integration, was replaced by new forms of leisure - or, in the case of women, by the overload of duties. While Pedro spent more time on activities such as watching TV and playing video games, and even taking occasional short walks outside, Ana and Sueli, both married, hardly found any free time while taking care of their children. "Since I have a 4-year-old daughter, she has been very demanding during this period because she isn't going to school", Ana confessed, "so I can't give her proper attention, nor to my work, nor to my master's degree, so everything becomes 'compartmentalised'".

The respondents were then asked whether they considered the fact that they are immigrants enhanced or reduced some of the reported impacts of the pandemic. For Carlos, immigrant status is not a problem in its own right, but rather the renewed social exclusion that these individuals may feel. "I don't believe that the pandemic hit immigrants more because they are immigrants", he explained, "but because they sometimes faced greater difficulties in being fully integrated into the system." This resulted in a lack of access to immigrant's rights, especially in cases where the immigrant's legalisation process is taking place after entering the country, which places the individual in what Carlos called a "legal limbo".

Despite this discourse, these immigrants felt an overall atmosphere of insecurity. As Cohen points out (2020), the sense of the lack of security felt by migrants during a pandemic can be revealed in many ways and in different dimensions, including a response to the fear of loss. In fact, insecurity was a recurring theme mentioned by the respondents. It soon became clear that the insecurity felt during the new COVID-19 pandemic did not derive from the immigrant status itself, but from what this condition represents in the individual's life. It was a perceived feeling of isolation referring to "not having anyone here, in case something happens", as Beatriz (30), a psychologist who has been living in Lisbon since 2019, explained, when "[...] you don't have, let's say, someone to count on. Nobody knows you; nobody is going to do anything for you. So, you're on your own." This feeling of insecurity was also portrayed as being far from family, friends, and from a common past that supports a linkage between the immigrant and the community of origin. "The feeling of being at home and of importance and insecurity for being an immigrant, is precisely not having my family around", said Carla, "so you end up not having the affection of your family members, the security of being within the family". Júlia described this as her "warmth", that meant "being close to 'my people'". For her, the realisation that everything could change at any moment intensified this feeling of wanting to be close to her family. "And sometimes you think 'no, I will withstand this moment, it will soon be over and everything will go back to normal.'", she said, "we can't think like that, because you blink and everything has changed, the world has changed." When we asked her to explain what she meant when she referred to her "cosiness", she told us: "the place that brings me security, the place where my children are, where my friends are, where are the people that I have lived my whole life."

In the words of Karine, insecurity is a way to describe the feeling of the Portuguese community in an economic scenario of instability, in which the search for job opportunities becomes more intense, when it is necessary to "compete" with immigrants. "Their insecurity is turning into hatred [...] and I would say mainly against Brazilians", she confessed. "I don't see the same prejudice against Angolans, for example, or Cape Verdeans, for example". This scenario is a consequence of processes of social comparison and perceived competition between groups in a situation of scarcity of resources, whereby the "Other" is seen as a threat, resulting in competitive behaviour (Campbell, 1965) that can be converted into situations of social discrimination and xenophobia. Such competition is exacerbated when there are social status asymmetries (Cf. Tajfel & Turner, 1979), which this helps us understand the rivalry mentioned by Karine: when the perceived social status of different nationalities of immigrants are assessed by Portuguese, those of African origin figure at the bottom of the perceived hierarchy, while Brazilians figure higher (Cabecinhas, 2007). The importance of the asymmetries of perceived social status was corroborated by Karine, when she explained the meaning she gives to this perceived competition: "They see Brazilians as being a little superior to them, although they don't admit it."

That's why, according to her, "they feel a bit more vulnerable. And then, to conceal this, they try to diminish us [Brazilians]".

After ascertaining the current impacts of the pandemic, we also decided to analyse its possible implications on plans for the future. Respondents were asked whether they have made any alterations to their life plans for the short or long term. It is interesting to note that the respondents who mentioned some change are those who have been in Portugal for the longest time, while for those who have migrated more recently, have kept their plans with few changes. In our survey, 10 out of 12 respondents who migrated in 2019 and 2020 said that the pandemic did not impact their future plans, while 6 out of 7 of those who migrated between 2016 and 2018 answered affirmatively to the question. This difference corroborates the statement by Castles and Miller (1998) that the very experience of migration and daily life in another place means that the original plans may be modified. This could explain why those who have lived longer in Portugal have had more time and experience in the new country to re-evaluate their plans, while newcomers have not yet had sufficient time to make such an evaluation. We also found that, for those who have lived in Portugal for longer, there was a higher feeling of uncertainty about the future, a characteristic of pandemic times and also the migratory journey itself.

Despite these differences, for those who claimed their plans have changed, the pandemic seems to have been interpreted as an invitation to reflect on personal goals over the short and long term. Some immigrants referred to it as a great pause in life, in which they took the opportunity to assess the pros and cons of the choices they have made in the past and which they must make in the future. "The pandemic, in some way, made me reflect on some issues that I had already thought about and that became stronger", commented Marina (34), an unemployed single Brazilian who has just returned from an Erasmus study period in Madrid to the North of Portugal, and intends to give up the master's degree that she started in Portugal to look for a job and thereby "guarantee a minimum income [economically speaking], if things get tight". For those who were already looking for a job, however, "the pandemic dashed our expectations", as Júlia said. She was the only respondent who stated she intended to return to Brazil because of the COVID-19 pandemic, since she admitted she had lost hope that she will be able to put herself in the job market during the pandemic or in the near future, which has led her to assess whether it is really worth staying in Portugal in her current conditions. She, therefore, decided that she will return to Brazil as soon as she can - a decision that was influenced by the "burden" of being away from her family. "The pandemic made me think, you know?", she said, "that I wanted to be close to those I always lived with, that I have always lived with, [those] who are 'mine': my family, my children, my brothers, my friends".

Except for Júlia, the other respondents have no intention of migrating once again or returning to Brazil. This discovery counters the notion that there is an increased intention to return to Brazil observed throughout the different migratory flows from Brazil to Portugal (Barbosa & Lima, 2020). This absence of changes indicates immigrants who, unlike those from other migratory waves, are planning to stay for longer in Portugal. "The plans remain the same", said Pedro. "I didn't come to take a rain check or anything, I came to change, to immigrate", he added. We noted that the matter, therefore, involves "waiting for the world to return to normal and continuing our life here", as Rodrigo (57), a retired doctor who moved to Aveiro this year, said. Something that "maybe changed the deadlines", according to Beatriz, of the plans mentioned by our respondents: buying a house, trying to find some part-time work, rescheduling the professional career or even bringing the family to live with them. Everything will depend, it appears, on the financial impact that the pandemic will have on these immigrants' lives. "I just need to know whether the financial impact is not going to be so severe that it obliges me to return", Pedro said.

Conclusions

Aiming to understand the impacts of the COVID-19 pandemic on the lives of recent Brazilian immigrants in Portugal, 19 of these individuals were interviewed in the months of May and June of 2020. Their responses were then submitted to a thematic analysis.

In relation to the impacts of the COVID-19 pandemic on their lives, the respondents recognised that the situation affected several different areas. Besides the impact on their economic status and the fear of unemployment, our research findings point to the fact that their daily routine and mental health were also affected. Gender inequalities and the matter of immigrant insecurity were also identified in our research, making it possible to understand that dealing with the pandemic is related to new leisure options and routine adjustments, and also an excessive burden of domestic tasks for women and the uncertainties and insecurities about insertion in the job market. Some of the immigrants interviewed mentioned cases of social discrimination in their professional environment related to their nationality, that can be related to scapegoating processes that are common in epidemics. Several respondents who said that the fact that they are immigrants does not influence the impact of the pandemic on their lives, explained that this is because they are in a privileged position in relation to other Brazilian immigrants who have directly faced adversities during the pandemic in Portugal. Another research finding is the reactivation of contact networks with Brazilians as a way to cope with the pandemic, which leads to the conclusion that contacts with those who remained in the origin country intensified, to the point of redeeming old affective relationships previously suppressed as a result of time and distance, frequently adopting a characteristic of care and monitoring of the situation of family and friends. Even so, this adverse scenario did not change the future plans of those who have migrated more recently, but imposed new schedules and deadlines for implementation of the life plans that they had drawn up before the pandemic.

Although these findings cannot be generalised to all Brazilian immigrants in Portugal, we believe that this study reveals several nuances that reflect broader social issues, synthesising several important points that deserve to be addressed in further studies on this topic.

Acknowledgement

We would like to thank the Brazilian immigrants who, during the challenging times we are all facing during this new COVID-19 pandemic, responded to our public call and dedicated some of their time to take part in this research.

References

Allport, G. W. (1954). *The nature of prejudice*. Cambridge: Addison-Wesley.

Barbosa, A., & Lima, A. (2020). *Brasileiros em Portugal: de volta às raízes lusitanas*. Brasília: Fundação Alexandre de Gusmão.

Cabecinhas, R. (2007). Preto e Branco: a naturalização da discriminação racial. Porto: Campo das Letras.

Campbell, D. (1965). "Ethnocentric and other altruistic motives". In: D. Levine (ed.) *Nebraska Symposium on Motivation*. Lincoln: University of Nebraska.

Campos, L. P., & Lins, T. (2020). "Pandemia à Portuguesa: um relato sobre o Covid-19 em Portugal", *Revista brasileira de geografia econômica*, 17. https://doi.org/10.4000/espacoeconomia.10369

Carvalhais, I. (2008). "Imigração e interculturalidade na União Europeia. Sombra e luz de uma relação complexa". In: R. Cabecinhas & L. Cunha (ed.) *Comunicação intercultural: Perspectivas, dilemas e desafios*. Porto: Campo das Letras.

Castles, S., & Miller, M. J. (1998). The Age of Migration: International Population Movements in the Modern World. London: MacMillan Press.

Chaiça, I. (2020, January 7). "Uma estranha forma de pneumonia está a preocupar a China. Causa é desconhecida", *Público*. https://www.publico.pt/2020/01/07/ciencia/noticia/estranha-forma-pneumonia-preocupar-china-causa-desconhecia-1899502

Cohen, J. (2020). "Modeling Migration, Insecurity and COVID-19", *Migration Letters*, 17 (3). https://doi.org/10.33182/ml.v17i3.986

Filho, A. (2020, March 23). "Brasileiros em Portugal e o vírus que lhes trouxe o desemprego", *Diário de Notícias*. https://www.dn.pt/pais/brasileiros-em-portugal-entre-a-ameaca-do-desemprego-e-o-medo-da-infecao-11971609.html

França, T., & Padilla, B. (2018). "Imigração Brasileira para Portugal: entre o surgimento e a construção mediática de uma nova vaga", *Cadernos de Estudos Sociais*, 33 (2): 207–237.

Francisco, J. (2020, May 6). "Bruxelas antecipa tombo de 6,8 % na economia portuguesa em 2020", *Diário de Notícias*. https://www.dn.pt/dinheiro/bruxelas-portugal-com-recessao-de-68-defice-de-65-e-a-sombra-do-turismo-12158811.html

Gaskell, G. (2003). "Entrevistas individuais e grupais". In: M. W. Bauer & G. Gaskell (eds.) *Pesquisa qualitativa com texto, imagem e som: um manual prático* (P. A. Guareschi, Trad.). Petrópolis: Vozes.

Glick, P. (2005). "Choice of Scapegoats". In: J. Dovidio, P. Glick and L. Rudman (eds.) *On the Nature of Prejudice: Fifty Years after Allport*. Oxford: Blackwell Publishing.

Hoppe, T. (2018). "'Spanish Flu': When Infectious Disease Name Blur Origins and Stigmatize Those Infected", *American Journal of Public Health*, 108 (11): 1462-1464. https://doi.org/10.2105/AJPH.2018.304645

INE. (2020). *Taxa de desemprego (Série 2011 - %) por Sexo, Grupo etário e Nível de escolaridade mais elevado completo; Trimestral.* https://ine.pt/xportal/xmain?xpid=INE&xpgid=ine_indicadores&contecto=pi&indOcorrCod=0005599&selTab=tab0

Lechner, E. (2007). "Imigração e saúde mental", *Revista Migrações - Número Temático Imigração e Saúde,* 1: 79-101. https://www.om.acm.gov.pt/documents/58428/1838 63/migracoes1_art4.pdf

Machado, I. (2014). "O futuro do passado: imigrantes brasileiros em Portugal e diferentes entrelaçamentos", *REMHU - Revista Interdisciplinar de Mobilidade Humana*, 43: 225-234. http://doi.org/10.1590/1980-85852503880004314

Ornell, F., Schuch, J.B., Sordi, A. O., Kessler, F.H.P. (2020). "'Pandemic fear' and COVID-19: mental health burden and strategies", *Brazilian Journal of Psychiatry*, 42 (3): 232-235. https://doi.org/10.1590/1516-4446-2020-0008

Padilla, B., Marques, J., Góis, P., & Peixoto, J. (2015). "A imigração brasileira em Portugal". In: J. Peixoto, B. Padilla, J. Marques and P. Góis (eds.) *Vagas Atlânticas: Migrações entre Brasil e Portugal no início do século XXI*. Lisbon: Mundos Sociais.

Páez, D., & Pérez, J. (2020). "Social representations of COVID-19", *International Journal of Social Psychology*. https://doi.org/10.1080/02134748.2020.1783852

SEF. (2010). *Relatório de Imigração, Fronteiras e Asilo 2009*. https://sefstat.sef.pt/Docs/Rifa_2009.pdf

SEF. (2020). *Relatório de Imigração, Fronteiras e Asilo 2019*. https://sefstat.sef.pt/Docs/Rifa2019.pdf

Severo, V. S. (2020). "Sobre a covid-19 e as nossas escolhas". In: A. Tostes and H. Filho (eds.) *Quarentena: reflexões sobre a pandemia e depois*. Bauru: Canal 6. [Kindle version]

Smith, N., O'Connor, C., & Joffe, H. (2015). "Social Representations of Threatening Phenomena: The Self-Other Thema and Identity Protection", *Papers on Social Representations*, 24 (2): 1.1–1.23.

Sobral, J., & Lima, M. (2018). "A epidemia pneumónica em Portugal no seu tempo histórico", *Ler História*, 73. https://doi.org/10.4000/lerhistoria.4036

Tajfel, H., & Turner, J. (1979). "An Integrative Theory of Intergroup Conflict". In: W. Austin and S. Worchel (eds.) *Psychology of intergroup relations*. Chicago: Nelson-Hall.

Talbot, M. (2007). *Media Discourse: representation and interaction*. Edinburgh: Edinburgh University Press.

Tracy, S. J. (2020). Qualitative Research Methods: Collecting Evidence, Crafting Analysis, Communicating Impact. New Jersey: Wiley Blackwell.

Vala, J., & Pereira, C. (2020). "Immigrants and Refugees: From Social Disaffection to Perceived Threat". In: D. Jodelet, J. Vala and E. Drozda-Senkowska (eds.) *Societies Under Threat: a Pluri-Disciplinary Approach*. New York: Springer.

Varennes, F. (2020). "COVID-19 fears should not be exploited to attack and exclude minorities – UN expert", *United Nations Human Rights Office of the High Comissioner*. https://www.ohchr.org/EN/NewsEvents/Pages/DisplayNews.aspx?NewsID=257 57

Waldron, T. (2020, May 20). "Brazil Is The New Epicenter Of The Global Coronavirus

Pandemic", *HuffPost*. https://www.huffpost.com/entry/bolsonaro-brazil-coronavirus-pandemic_n_5ec5662ac5b6dcbe36022e5a

WHO. (2020, March 12). "WHO announces COVID-19 outbreak a pandemic", *World Health Organization*. http://www.euro.who.int/en/health-topics/health-emergencies /coronavirus-covid-19/news/news/2020/3/who-announces-covid-19-outbreak-a-pandemic

CHAPTER 11

MIGRATION AND IMMIGRATION: UGANDA AND THE COVID-19 PANDEMIC

Agnes Igoye

Introduction

This is a reflective commentary on the changing nature of Border Management in Uganda amidst the COVID-19 crisis. The COVID-19 pandemic is the largest health and mobility crisis that our world has ever seen. Following travel restrictions and lock-downs, several countries are gradually opening their air spaces; however, border Governance will never be the same. To restore confidence in global travel, countries will have to rethink their Border Governance regimes, structures, protocols and procedures to accommodate health safety COVID-19 guidelines

My first confrontation with a border management crisis was in 2007-08, during my tenure as a border guard at the Uganda-Kenya Busia border. The crisis erupted after former President Mwai Kibaki was declared the winner of the Presidential election in Kenya. The opposition, led by Raila Odinga of the Orange Democratic Movement, alleged election manipulation. As the New York Times reported then: "With the president, Mwai Kibaki, a Kikuyu and Mr Odinga a Luo, the election seems to have tapped into an atavistic vein of tribal tension that always lay beneath the surface in Kenya but until now had not provoked widespread mayhem" (NYT, 2007).

As many international organizations, including humanitarian organizations and embassies, issued travel advisories for their workers and nationals to evacuate, I was among the border guards taking cover from bullets, stones and machetes while rescuing fleeing Kenyans and migrants, many of whom were wounded seeking protection across the border.

Prior to this, I had faced another incident at the same border in 2006 when I confronted and caused the arrest of one of the Lord's Resistance Army's (LRA) notorious commanders. He had killed people in Northern Uganda, forcing villagers to cook and eat human flesh. In the process, my colleagues and I rescued the women and young girls that the LRA rebels had abducted as sex slaves (New Vision, 2006).

These two incidences highlight political and civil unrest, and we had structures for addressing it. Conversely, when the COVID-19 pandemic struck, it was an invisible enemy, one that caused unique global panic. Countries shut down and border closures ensued as a measure for countries to safeguard their nationals from the pandemic. I was among the essential workers based at the COVID-19 Situation room in Uganda, monitoring national borders at the Directorate of Citizenship and Immigration Control.

Here is what I learned during my weeks of intensive work to keep Uganda safe by focusing on borders:

Cross-border Movements During Lock-downs

In many countries, border closures could not complete insulate people from the spread of disease as it did not mean no one crossed the border. This was the case in Uganda, which has a colonial legacy where the arbitrary partition of Africa left unclear border demarcations. Border communities and families were separated, and now a legacy of porous borders remains. Irregular border crossings are utilized by these cross-border communities to keep connected. Transnational organized criminals have also leveraged these irregular border crossings for their illegal activities, including trafficking in persons, drugs and arms. This is not unique to Uganda, but a common scenario in Africa and globally, and it continued even during the COVID-19 lockdowns.

Irregular Migrants

The exclusion of migrant workers and victims of human trafficking from COVID-19 interventions has pushed many migrants further into irregular situations, forcing some of them to use irregular border crossings despite lock-downs and restrictions of movement.

In my interactions with guards at Uganda's borders with Kenya, one category of people using irregular routes during lock-downs are Migrant domestic workers. In most cases, these workers are in the informal economy. This gives them poor legal protection, and they are excluded from labour rights and social security safety nets. Their Exclusion is particularly linked to certain characteristics: irregular status, unpredictable income and work time, working with multiple employers and as live-in workers.

They are among the migrant workers often excluded from national COVID-19 policy responses, such as wage subsidies, unemployment benefits, social security and social protection measures. Compared to nationals, migrant workers are often the last to gain access to testing or treatment. In the case of domestic workers, exclusion from social security and COVID-19 related support is derived from the fact that most national labour laws do not regard them as workers (ILO, 2020).

Tighter restrictions on unskilled labour migration in many countries have driven low-skilled migrants to irregular ways of migration, making them vulnerable to exploitation. They will not seek redress, for fear of job loss, deportation or incarceration

Except for migrants trapped overseas who can only use a flight to return, some migrants from neighbouring countries risk it all by traversing irregular routes to avoid border patrol. Loss of income and layoffs of migrant workers has led to the expiration of visa or work permits, putting migrants into irregular status. For instance, when Kenya relaxed its lock-down, there was a spike of the number of people apprehended for using irregular crossings and taken to Uganda's Ministry of Health designated centers for the mandatory 14 days quarantine.

Refugees and Asylum Seekers

The COVID-19 pandemic, and subsequent restrictions on the movement of persons, collided with other crises around Africa, causing forced migration. Specifically, these crises include Climate disaster such as drought, landslides, floods and locust plagues, as well as civil/political instability (DW, 2020).

For a country like Uganda, known for its generous and progressive refugee policies, this shift caused President Yoweri Museveni to direct temporal reopening of Uganda's borders between July 1-3, to allow over 3,000 refugees from the Democratic Republic of the Congo (DRC) to enter the country (UNHCR, 2020a).

Uganda's border management procedures had to be changed, requiring new arrivals to undergo a 14-day mandatory quarantine before their transportation to existing refugee settlements, in line with national COVID-19 guidelines and protocols. The United Nations High Commission for Refugees (UNHCR) applauded Uganda's efforts "as an example of how careful border management can respect international human rights and refugee protection standards amid the pandemic." (UNHCR, 2020b)

COVID-19 infections from imported cases among refugees remains a challenge. According to UNHCR COVID-19 Response Bi-Monthly Update, out of 1,425,040 refugees and asylum seekers (as of June 2020), 52 tested positive to COVID-19, 52 refugees recovered while 2,919 refugees and asylum seekers are in quarantine.

A coordinated regional response is needed to safeguard displaced persons, asylum seekers, refugees and host communities from the spread of pandemics (ReliefWeb, 2020).

Emphasis on Migration and Health

When the COVID-19 pandemic was declared, no country was fully prepared, and little was known about the disease. In Uganda, the capacity of the health sector to secure the borders was limited and had to be enhanced. The situation is better today but has brought in new challenges.

The emphasis on managing the pandemic has hindered effective response to other forms of transnational organized crimes like human trafficking. In Uganda, while the borders remain closed, people who have been found using porous/irregular routes are placed on compulsory 14-day quarantine. In my routine interactions with border guards, since persons are taken straight for isolation, they are unable to interview them, identify possible victims of human trafficking for adequate protection services, nor identify their traffickers.

Integrated Border Management

The COVID-19 Pandemic teaches some lessons to ensure effective border governance. Integrated border management is key to unlocking disjointedness in border Governance. According to the International Organization for Migration (IOM), "Integrated Border Management requires that all competent authorities work together in an effective and efficient manner" (IOM, 2015).

As COVID-19 has taught us, agencies responsible for migration health cannot work in isolation during a pandemic, or simply wait for a pandemic to happen to include health Ministries and agencies in border management. Interdisciplinary agencies should work collectively and sustainably under the integrated border management arrangement.

The African Union (AU) Convention on Cross Border Cooperation (Niamey Convention, 2012) aims to ensure efficient and effective integrated border management – specifically in Article 2(5). The convention also stipulates the principle and instrument of cross border cooperation (CBC), defined as: "any act or policy aimed at promoting and strengthening good neighbour relations between border populations, territorial communities and administrations or other stakeholders within the jurisdiction of two or more states, including the conclusion of agreement useful for this purpose." (UN, 2018).

A corporation under integrated border management should be established both within the specific country, as well as across borders with relevant agencies of neighbouring states. As IOM stipulates: "[the agency] should seek to address three levels of cooperation and coordination: intra-service cooperation, inter-agency cooperation and international cooperation." (IOM,

2015).

In times of calm, stakeholders responsible for border governance should be involved in perfecting their levels of preparedness. This can be done through creating and strengthening early warning systems, coordination mechanisms, building infrastructure, human resource development/training front-line officers, enhancing migration intelligence capabilities, research and policy work.

For instance, the Inter-Governmental Authority on Development (IGAD) member states established a Conflict Early Warning and Response Mechanism (CEWARN) in 2002. However, this is mainly geared toward preventing violent conflicts. For an adequate regional response to pandemics and disease, a sustainable early warning health system should be developed. This would enable adequate preparedness and quick sharing of information concerning disease and pandemics to prevent further outbreak and escalation (CEWARN, 2020).

Further lessons can be drawn from the International Organization for Migration (IOM's) Health, Border & Mobility Management (HBMM) conceptual and operational framework. The framework aims at improving prevention, detection and response to the spread of diseases at national points of origin, transit, destination and return. Interventions extend to Spaces of vulnerability, where migrants and mobile populations interact with stationary, local communities. With a particular focus on border areas, HBMM unifies border management with health security and ultimately supports the implementation of the 2005 International Health Regulations (IHR) (IOM, 2020).

One-Stop-Border-Post (OSBPs)

One aspect of integrated border management is a One-Stop-Border-Post (OSBPs) model. This has been implemented in various capacities and regions, and is a single, shared physical infrastructure in which the neighbouring countries' customs and border services operate side by side. In Uganda, there are currently five OSBPs, some of which did not have a consistent presence of an agency responsible for migration health prior to the pandemic. Sustainable presence of the health agencies would facilitate adequate inter agency collaboration and coordination under the integrated border management dispensation (IOM, 2015).

Border Communities

Social mobilization, population awareness and instilling behaviour change is not easy but critical during a pandemic. Even more challenging is when cross border communities and families are expected to stay at home, separated from their loved ones who live on both sides of an international border. The colonial legacy of border demarcations created constant border disputes across Africa, but also separated families and communities. Instilling restrictions of movement across land borders is particularly challenging where irregular border crossings exist. This fact, compounded with inadequate access to information due to limited or lack of internet and smartphones during lock-down, complicates the challenge.

Uganda's experience responding to Ebola provided valuable lessons. The local council (LC) system of governance proved to be an effective local mobilization tool. Traditional roles of these local leaders include: handling land and civil disputes governed by customary law, assaults and battery and trespass and property damages cases. Apart from this, these local leaders provided leadership in community awareness before, during and after a crisis. They live within and know their communities better (New Vision, nd).

In my own community, I was involved with our Local council 1 (LC1) chairman in mobilizing resources to feed the people who lacked food during lock-down. Support to migrants and mobile populations, as well as host communities, notably those residing along borders and in migrant-dense areas, is critical to limit their cross-border movements in search for essential commodities/ food in shared markets, gardens and other shared economic and social spaces.

Limiting border communities from accessing cross border shared spaces such as markets and houses of worship reduces the risk of spread of pandemics across borders. The local council system has worked for Uganda. While guarding against xenophobia and discrimination, LC's have sensitized their communities that have become vigilant and mindful of any visitors to their communities during a pandemic.

Need for enhanced technology and Database Integration

I was part of the essential staff at the Directorate of Citizenship and Immigration Control (DCIC) Situation room during total lock-down of the COVID-19 response in Uganda. One of our activities was coordinating and collecting regular information, including daily updates from Uganda's 54 gazetted border stations and Uganda's 336 porous borders. This process was tedious and time consuming. It involved making phone calls, using email, social media and constantly diligently recording all information. Information was then manually analyzed and shared with various agencies like the Ministry of Health and the National COVID-19 taskforce.

A disjointed, unintegrated border management system is a deterrent to quick decision making, sharing of information and missed opportunities for interagency collaboration. This is especially evident during a pandemic, where limited human contact and social distancing is the working standard.

Investing in Integrated information technology systems, infrastructure, and staff training is a prerequisite for effective Migration Governance. It facilitates fast, real time interagency sharing of information for quick decision making (UN, 2018).

The Declarations of the African Union Border Programme and its Implementation Modalities, adopted by the Conference of African Ministers in Charge of Border Issues (2007, 2010 and 2012), stress the need to put in place a new form of pragmatic border management system aimed at promoting peace, security and stability, as well as facilitating the integration process and sustainable development in Africa. Given the current challenges in border management due to the COVID-19 Pandemic, a holistic approach that equally prioritizes Issues of Migration health should be part of this agenda.

Border Patrol Capabilities

Uganda is a landlocked nation, with 53 staffed and over 336 unstaffed (porous) irregular border crossings as of July 2020. Uganda's long and complex land border of 2729 kilometers is shared with five other countries: DRC, Kenya, Rwanda, South Sudan, and Tanzania (CIA, nd).

Porous borders are not unique to Africa, but are a global challenge faced by many countries. Well-established, professional border patrol units are a prerequisite for effective border control during a pandemic. Their training should extend beyond curbing irregular migration and transnational organized crime. It must include Migration health training and equipping frontline officers to protect countries/border communities against cross border spread of disease. If countries had had better trained frontline/border patrol officers, cross border spread of COVID-19 would have been minimized. Free Movement in Persons Regimes In late February 2020, as countries began instilling restrictions of movement to contain the COVID-19 pandemic, I was in Sudan, as part of the Inter-Governmental Authority on Development (IGAD) team of expert negotiators of the Protocol on Free Movement of Persons in the IGAD Region. IGAD Member States with more than 230 million people, covers an area of over 5.2 million km2 that comprises the countries of Djibouti, Eritrea, Ethiopia, Kenya, Somalia, South Sudan, Sudan and Uganda (IGAD, 2016).

While in Sudan, we had concluded negotiations to the Free Movement of Persons protocol and witnessed its endorsement. Congratulating the eight Member States led by their Ministers in charge of Internal Affairs and those in charge of Labor, IGAD's Executive Secretary Dr Workneh acknowledged that "the Protocol was a major milestone on our journey towards peace, prosperity & ultimately regional and continental integration."

As the architects of the Migration Policy Framework for Africa and Plan of Action (2018-2020) warned, the trend towards the securitization of migration and borders should not engender the closing of borders and hamper integration efforts in Africa (UN, 2018).

With the advent of COVID-19, countries have to lay down safeguards to secure borders from the spread of pandemics, to restore confidence to actualize free movement regimes. The implementation of the Continental Free Trade Area (CFTA) and the AU Free Movement of Persons Regimes Protocol will rely on progress made towards securing Africa's borders from the disease. This will require harmonization of health border procedures, policies and laws, transnational cooperation and information sharing among authorities responsible for Migration/border Governance.

References

CEWARN (2020). CEWARN. https://www.cewarn.org/index.php/about-cewarn. Accessed: 1/4/2020.

CIA (nd). CIA World Factbook – Uganda. https://www.cia.gov/library/publications/the-world-factbook/geos/ug.html. Accessed: 1/4/2020.

DW (2020). Uganda Remains steadfast on refugees. *Deutsche Welle.* Available: https://www.dw.com/en/uganda-remains-steadfast-on-refugees-despite-covid-19/a-54041165. Accessed: 1/4/2020.

IGAD (2016). IGAD. https://igad.int/divisions/health-and-social-development/2016-05-24-03-16-37/2373-protocol-on-free-movement-of-persons-endorse-at-ministerial-meeting and https://igad.int/about-us/the-igad-region. Accessed: 1/4/2020.

ILO (2018). 2018 ILO skills for employment policy brief. Available: https:/ILO%20eSSAY/Policy%20Brief_Skills.pdf. Accessed: 1/4/2020.

ILO (2020). 2020 ILO Policy brief. Available: https://www.ilo.org/wcmsp5/groups/public/---ed_protect/---protrav/---migrant/documents/publication/wcms_743268.pdf. Accessed: 1/4/2020.

IOM (2015). https://www.iom.int/sites/default/files/our_work/DMM/IBM/updated/05_FACT_SHEET_Integrated_Border_Management_2015.pdf. Accessed: 1/4/2020.

IOM (2020). https://www.iom.int/sites/default/files/our_work/DMM/IBM/2020/en/en_covid-19ibmresponseinfosheet_2pages.pdf. Accessed: 1/4/2020.

New Vision (nd). New Vision LC 1 Chairperson. https://www.newvision.co.ug/news/1481237/exactly-role-lc1-chairperson. Accessed: 1/4/2020.

New Vision (2006). 2006 LRA Border Arrest, *New Vision.* Available: https://www.newvision.co.ug/news/1145793/kony-eur-wife-netted-busia-border. Accessed: 1/4/2020.

NYT (2007). Kenyan Election Conflict. *New York Times.* Available: https://www.nytimes.com/2007/12/31/world/africa/31kenya.html Accessed: 1/4/2020.

ReliefWeb (2020). https://reliefweb.int/report/uganda/uganda-unhcr-covid-19-response-bi-monthly-update-6-july-2020. Accessed: 1/4/2020.

UN (2018). 2018 Migration Policy Framework for Africa). Available: https://violenceagainstchildren.un.org/sites/violenceagainstchildren.un.org/files/documents/other_documents/35316-doc-au-mpfa_2018-eng.pdf. Accessed: 1/4/2020.

UNHCR (2020a). UNHCR Data. Available: https://data2.unhcr.org/en/documents/download/64687. Accessed: 1/4/2020.

UNHCR (2020b). UNHCR Reporting. Available: https://reporting.unhcr.org/sites/default/files/UNHCR%20EHAGL%20COVID-19%20EXTERNAL%20update%20%2315.pdf

CHAPTER 12

IMPACT OF COVID-19 HUMAN MOBILITY RESTRICTIONS ON THE MIGRANT ORIGIN POPULATION IN FINLAND

Natalia Skogberg, Idil Hussein and Anu E Castaneda

Introduction

Finland is a Northern European country, bordering with Norway, Sweden and Russia. The total population is 5,5 million. Up until the 1990s, Finland has been mainly a country of emigration. Since then, however, the size of the migrant origin population grew from half per cent to approximately eight per cent in 2019 (OSF 2020a). The largest migrant origin groups residing in Finland are from Russia and the former Soviet Union, Estonia, Sweden, Iraq and Somalia. Migration has concentrated particularly towards the Helsinki metropolitan area, with half of the migrant population residing in this region (OSF 2020b). The main reasons for migration to Finland are family reunification, employment and studies, with a substantially lower proportion of persons arriving as resettlement refugees or asylum seekers (Ministry of the Interior 2019).

With a record low birth rate over the past years, migration is currently the main reason for population growth in Finland. Migration is also necessary for the national economic growth and development, particularly in the light of the rapid ageing of the Finnish-born population. The age structure of the migrant origin population is substantially younger compared with that of Finnish origin. By the end of 2019, approximately a quarter of the Finnish origin population had reached retirement age (65 years and older), whereas the respective proportion in the migrant origin population was six per cent (OSF 2020a).

Over the recent years, the Finnish Government has made legislative and policy changes to further attract work and student-based migration and to lower the barriers for entering the labour market of migrants already residing in Finland (Ministry of the Interior 2019). In addition to providing highly-specialised expertise and acting as entrepreneurs, migrants significantly contribute to filling the labour shortage in a variety of manual professions within the construction, agriculture, catering and hospitality, cleaning, healthcare and transport industries (Sutela 2015; Ministry of the Interior 2019). In addition to those migrating to Finland with the purpose of resettling, the migrant labour force in Finland also constitutes of seasonal workers and EU country nationals who travel to Finland for shorter periods of time.

The aim of this chapter is to describe the changes in human mobility as the result of the COVID-19 pandemic in Finland and to discuss the consequences of these measures on the health and wellbeing of persons of migrant origin in Finland. First, the strategy of the Finnish Government for dealing with the COVID-19 pandemic and the restrictions on human mobility are described. Second, the best available information to date on the incidence of COVID-19 among the migrant origin population in Finland is presented. Third, the consequences for migration patterns and the health, economic situation and psychosocial wellbeing of persons of migrant origin are discussed.

This text is based on research findings, press releases by various authorities, reliable media sources and exchanges with various experts working in the field of migration as well as with the representatives of the migrant origin populations themselves. The writers are experts in multicultural issues at the Finnish Institute for Health and Welfare (THL) and are involved in evaluating the effects of COVID-19 on the health and wellbeing of persons of migrant origin. This text covers the situation in Finland up to the middle of July 2020. How the COVID-19 situation evolves in Finland following this period remains to be seen.

COVID-19 and human mobility in Finland

The first case of COVID-19 in Finland was observed at the end of January 2020, when a tourist from China was diagnosed with the virus shortly after arrival to Northern Finland. This remained a single case until the end of February, when Finnish nationals returning from travels in Northern Italy were diagnosed with COVID-19. Despite quarantine regulations, effective tracking of potentially contaminated persons and dissemination of information on preventive measures by the health authorities, COVID-19 spread in the Finnish population.

Based on lessons learned from other countries at further stages of the pandemic, Finland quickly introduced a set of restrictive measures based on health authority recommendations, legislations under normal conditions and the emergency power legislation. On March 16th 2020, the Finnish Government together with the President of the Republic declared a state of emergency in Finland over the COVID-19 outbreak. The Government submitted a decree for implementing the Emergency Powers Act to the Parliament the following day. The state of emergency lasted for three months. (Finnish Government 2020a)

During this period, a set of highly restrictive measures were introduced under the effect of the Emergency Powers Act. These included closing down of educational, cultural, sports and other recreational facilities. Kindergartens and lower primary school grades remained open, however parents were strongly advised to keep children at home. Gatherings of more than ten people were prohibited and spending time in public places was to be avoided. Persons aged 70 years or older were strongly advised to self-isolate and visits to assisted living facilities of elderly and other risk groups were prohibited. Visitations to hospitals and other healthcare facilities were also prohibited with several possible exemptions evaluated on case-by-case basis. (Finnish Government 2020a) Finland's international borders were closed to foreigners and non-residents. In addition to restricting international travel, the Government imposed restrictions on internal travel in the Southern Finland by closing the borders of the Uusimaa region for three weeks from the end of March until mid-April (Finnish Government 2020b). Intensive care capacity was doubled in order to meet the demands of COVID-19 care. The capacity for COVID-19 testing was gradually increased with the support from THL from 1,700 samples a day in mid-March to over 13,000 samples per day in June.

At the beginning of May, the growth of the coronavirus pandemic had been halted through restrictive measures and a clear improvement in hygiene behaviour and the Finnish Government decided to adopt a hybrid strategy for managing the COVID-19 crisis. The hybrid strategy focuses on a "test, trace, isolate and treat" approach, alongside a gradual dismantling of restrictive measures in order to minimize the adverse impact on people, businesses, society and the exercise of fundamental rights. From mid-May onwards, primary and secondary school students returned to classroom teaching and gatherings of 10 people were allowed. Restaurants, recreational facilities and libraries were cautiously opened with the condition that social distancing regulations were followed.

On June 15th, the Finnish Government declared that the current pandemic situation in Finland no longer fulfilled the criteria for the implementation of the Emergency Power Act (Finnish Government 2020c). Restrictions on human mobility from then on were regulated through various acts effective during normal conditions, such as the Communicable Diseases Act and other legislation under normal conditions. By the beginning of July, it was possible to hold public gatherings up to 500 persons. From mid-June, traveling to Finland from Norway, Denmark, Iceland, Estonia, Latvia and Lithuania was allowed without a two-week (voluntary) quarantine period.

From mid-July onwards, further alleviations were made in traveling from EU and Schengen countries as well as a number of other countries as long as the incidence of COVID-19 over the most recent 14 days remains below 8 cases per 100 000 persons. Despite these alleviations, traveling within Finland instead of international travel was highly recommended.

Consequences of COVID-19 and human mobility restrictions for migrants

Migration patterns

Migration to Finland practically stopped upon the closing of the Finnish borders. Under the Constitution of Finland, Finnish citizens always have the right to return to Finland. Simultaneously, everyone has the right to leave the country, provided that there is no legal impediment to this. We are not aware of estimates on how many foreign origin persons traveling abroad during the outbreak of the COVID-19 crisis were unable to return to Finland. Persons who were planning migration to Finland, whether it was as refugees, to work, study or for the purpose of family reunification, were not able to cross the Finnish border. The number of first-time asylum seekers diminished dramatically during the COVID-19 pandemic. Asylum interviews were temporally interrupted between mid-March to mid-April and only decisions for those who have already undergone the asylum interview were processed (Finnish Immigration Service 2020a).

Mobility restrictions caused substantial labour shortage in agriculture, which relies heavily on migrant seasonal workers. Under normal circumstances, an estimated 16,000 migrant seasonal workers work in agriculture (Loula 2020). By mid-June, the Finnish Immigration Service had granted a work permit for almost 9,000 persons from outside of EU (Finnish Immigration Service 2020b). By the beginning of July, however, only approximately 5,000 seasonal workers had arrived in Finland, mainly from Ukraine but also from the Baltic countries, including Romania and Bulgaria. While Finland is ready to receive seasonal workers also from outside of the EU, restrictions in the country of origin have made their arrival challenging (Heiskanen & Saatsi 2020).

Closing of the Finnish borders affected tens of thousands of Estonians regularly commuting between Finland and Estonia for work. They were faced with the decision whether they would stay to work in Finland separated from their families for an unknown period of time or whether they would return home to Estonia with no guarantee of a salary (Onali 2020).

An estimated 3,000 Finns cross the Finland-Sweden border daily for work (Ruokakangas 2020). With imposed border restrictions, work-related travel to Sweden became more complex, although traveling for essential work was still allowed. Quarantine of 14 days was expected from those crossing the border, with the exception for personnel in emergency medical service, rescue service and freight transport (The Border Guard organization 2020). The region in North-West Finland, where many Finns cross over to Sweden for work, has the highest incidence of COVID-19 outside of Helsinki and Uusimaa Health District. The proximity of the Swedish border is thought to be the cause of the high incidence rate (Ruokakangas 2020).

Closing of the Finnish border with Russia did not only cut-off Russian origin migrants (by far the largest migrant origin group in Finland) from traveling to visit their relatives in Russia, but also put an abrupt stop to travels of nearly 2 million Russian tourists to Finland each year. It is likely that the Finnish-Russian border will be among the last restrictive measures to be alleviated due to the substantially worse COVID-19 situation in Russia compared with Finland (Yle News 2020).

Health consequences

Incidence of COVID-19 among migrants

The COVID-19 incidence is monitored by the THL, working under the Ministry of Social Affairs and Health. THL advises the Government on containment measures based on this information. Despite the initially quite gloomy predictions, it appears that the measures taken by the Finnish Government to prevent the spread of COVID-19 were highly effective. By mid-July, there was a total of 7 296 COVID-19 cases and 328 deaths. Out of the detected cases, a substantial majority (73 %) were detected in the Helsinki metropolitan area. (THL 2020a)

Although the incidence of COVID-19 is not systematically published according to the country of origin, it has been reported that some migrant origin groups are overrepresented among the diagnosed cases. In particular, infections among the Somali origin population have been reported. By the middle of April, 1.8 per cent of the Somali population in Helsinki were tested positive for COVID-19, whereas the respective prevalence was 0.2 per cent in the Finnish origin population (Helsinki City Executive Office 2020). Overrepresentation of persons of migrant origin in the incidence of COVID-19 has also been reported in other countries, including Sweden (Public Health Agency of Sweden 2020), Norway (Norwegian Institute of Public Health), Britain (Platt & Warwick 2020) and the United States (CDC 2020).

The suggested reasons for a higher disease incidence among persons of migrant origin include crowded housing. Furthermore, migrants are more likely to live in multigenerational households, which increase the likelihood of older and more vulnerable persons becoming infected. Migrants may not have other options than using public transport to travel for work. Other proposed reasons include a high proportion of migrants in healthcare and overall in the service and transport industry, where people cannot avoid face-to-face contact with other people. Some migrant groups, in particular, have a higher incidence of chronic conditions, such as diabetes and obesity, which may predispose to complications related to COVID-19 (Skogberg et al. 2018, Skogberg et al. 2016).

Social and cultural factors may also influence the observed higher incidence of COVID-19 in some migrant origin groups. People may place different importance to social and physical connectedness. Religious leaders may have a great deal more authority than the Government or health authorities. In some religious circles, people may believe that the actions of individuals do not directly influence the spread of disease. (Saukkonen 2020)

Out of the 40 reception centres in Finland hosting approximately 7700 asylum seekers, only one reception centre in the metropolitan region has been severely affected by an outbreak of COVID-19 when nearly half of it's 300 residents were diagnosed with the virus (Finnish Immigration Service 2020c). This led to the testing of all the residents in this reception centre. Majority of the diagnosed cases were asymptomatic or with mild symptoms and none of the asylum seekers had to be hospitalised. The rest of the reception centres in Finland had only a few cases of COVID-19 and it was possible to contain these despite the generally crowded living conditions of asylum seekers.

Following alleviations to border control and some exceptions to regulations regarding seasonal workers, clusters of COVID-19 outbreaks among migrants at construction sites and among seasonal workers in agriculture were reported (THL 2020b, Loula 2020). The outbreaks were most likely related to crowded housing and insufficient hygiene. It was stressed that the employer is also responsible for ensuring adequate living conditions that allow for social distancing and ensuring that updated official recommendations by the health authorities reach the workers.

Improving adherence to recommendations through multilingual information

THL has been central also in disseminating information on COVID-19 among the Finnish population. Already at the start of the pandemic, it became evident that there was an acute demand for multilingual information and other coordination issues with respect to COVID-19 among the migrant origin population in Finland. To meet this demand, the Ministry of Social Affairs and Health and THL formed a task force to discuss and coordinate multilingual and multichannel communication for persons of migrant origin. The task force met on a weekly basis to monitor the situation and to discuss possible actions. Roundtable discussions were also held to share information bidirectionally with health and social service professionals from the Government and NGO sector as well as religious leaders and national minority professionals and influencers from migrant communities in Finland.

In total, THL produced multilingual instructions in 20 languages to better target the persons of migrant origin in March and in 13 languages in June 2020 (THL 2020c). The task force was also involved in production of Ramadan communication materials. THL produced social media materials and the task force contributed to video material produced by the Prime Minister's office and religious leaders from the Muslim community in Finland (THL 2020d, Finnish Government 2020d).

THL's expert group for cultural diversity (MONET) reached out to partners from the migration and cultural diversity field (including the Finnish Roma population) to collaborate in sharing of communication materials on COVID-19 as well as to discuss the impact of COVID-19 in the above-mentioned communities. Furthermore, THL worked together with the Finnish Immigration Service in the follow-up of the COVID-19 pandemic at the reception centre in the metropolitan area suffering from the major outbreak of the virus. THL also participated in a multidisciplinary network gathered by the city of Helsinki to discuss methods for prevention of the spread of COVID-19, especially among the Somali origin population.

From the experiences of the THL's task force, representatives of migrant communities and non-governmental organisations reported difficulties among persons of migrant origin in seeking healthcare, contact tracing and receiving adequate healthcare services. Some migrants sought out help from the healthcare services already at a very late stage of the disease. It is possible that this could be because of fear of stigmatisation or discrimination or insufficient understanding of recommendations regarding seeking care. According to the THL's task force observations, some difficulties were also experienced with regard to understanding and implementing the quarantine guidelines made by the healthcare professionals. It is likely that better availability of multilingual healthcare personnel and interpreters would have alleviated these difficulties at least partially.

Observations of the THL's task force are in line with the findings of a recent study focusing on Arabic, Somali and Russian-speaking migrants mainly aged 50 years and older. According to the preliminary findings, information on COVID-19 had reached the Russian and Somali-speaking population quite well, whereas the Arabic-speaking respondents had more difficulties in accessing reliable information. Persons of Somali origin were also better aware of which healthcare officials should be contacted if they suspected a COVID-19 infection (Finell, 2020).

The long-term impact of COVID-19 on the health of persons of migrant origin will be seen only in due course. While some have likely experienced positive lifestyle changes following the onset of restrictive measures of COVID-19 pandemic, many may have reduced their physical activity levels while caloric intake may have increased. Chronic disease risk factors, such as overweight and obesity and elevated glucose levels have been higher among some migrant origin groups in Finland already prior to the COVID-19 pandemic (Skogberg et al., 2018, Skogberg et al., 2016) and the prevalence of these may have further increased as a result of the pandemic.

Non-urgent healthcare services scheduled from mid-March to the end of April were postponed as healthcare personnel was transferred to work in tasks related to COVID-19. In addition to postponement of healthcare visits by the service providers, patients themselves cancelled a large proportion of their non-urgent appointments. The number of people seeking medical advice for other reasons than acute symptoms dropped dramatically. Even though the provision of non-urgent healthcare services was resumed from May onwards, use of these remained at a much lower level than prior to the pandemic (Parhiala & Jormanainen, 2020). This raised concerns that the timely diagnosis and treatment of chronic conditions have been delayed and people have been left without the needed supportive services. This, in turn, may have a detrimental effect on the health and wellbeing in the long run. Migrants in particular experience higher barriers in access to healthcare services under normal circumstances (Koponen et al., 2016) and the COVID-19 pandemic may have further exacerbated these.

Economic and psychosocial consequences

Unemployment rates and lay-offs increased dramatically as a consequence of substantial restrictions on the provision of private services, transportation and production of cultural and other recreational services. Especially people working in sales and the service industry were affected. Many migrants lost their jobs or have been laid off. If unemployment continues, this will impact the legal status of migrants who have been granted a temporal residence permit in Finland on the grounds of work. Unemployment also impacted the opportunities for family reunification due to the high financial eligibility threshold. Although international students were generally able to continue studying through distance learning, many have lost the part-time jobs that they relied upon to finance their studies (Saukkonen, 2020). The COVID-19 pandemic further weakened re-employment opportunities of the most vulnerable unemployed groups, including migrants, long-term unemployed, persons with long-term disabilities, and persons aged 50 years and older (Eronen et al., 2020).

The COVID-19 pandemic had a significant impact on integration processes of recent migrants. As was the case with other types of education, integration training was shifted to distance learning. It is likely that technical challenges, lack of adequate equipment and psychosocial stress related to COVID-19 have made learning more difficult at least for some recent migrants, affecting the smoothness of their integration process. Social distancing regulations have substantially decreased opportunities for social interaction and building of social networks, which are central for adapting to the new living environment. With a shift to distance learning, concerns have also been raised regarding an increase in already existing educational inequalities among different population groups, placing children and youth of migrant origin at a greater risk for social disadvantage (Saukkonen, 2020).

The consequences of the COVID-19 pandemic for the psychological wellbeing of the Finnish population have been widely discussed. The main perspectives relate to how to cope with the mental health problems and psychological burden (e.g. anxiety) that may be increased by the COVID-19 pandemic or the consequences of it, such as fear of oneself or a close one getting the virus or the financial downfalls caused by the pandemic. There is yet no information available on the mental health status of the migrant origin population in Finland during the COVID-19 pandemic. However, previous studies have shown a higher affective symptom prevalence in some migrant origin groups in comparison with the general population in Finland (Castaneda et al. 2020; Rask et al. 2016), thus making the mental health consequences of the COVID-19 among persons of migrant origin of particular concern.

According to the preliminary findings of a recent study, the majority of the interviewed Arabic, Somali and Russian-speaking respondents reported being at least somewhat concerned about the COVID-19 pandemic. Concerns were expressed with regard to own health and that of close ones, the situation in the country of origin, travel restrictions, own employment and financial situation, lack of a cure and vaccine for COVID-19, as well as the official's ability to deal with the crisis (ex. sufficiency of face masks). Excess of information on COVID-19 as well as doubts regarding the reliability of the information also raised concerns. Coping strategies included avoiding thinking of the pandemic, following official recommendations and taking good care of their own health, as well as faith in God (Finell 2020).

In some migrant populations, restrictions caused by COVID-19 have caused a great deal of worry to the families of those who have deceased during the pandemic. Around the world, funerals and burials take many forms, and the burial process can be very sensitive for the family and the community. Funerals hold particular importance and in some religions, it is mandatory to follow certain steps in the burial process. However, the COVID-19 pandemic has forced the world to re-think the entire process.

In order to counteract the detrimental psychosocial effects of COVID-19 on the wellbeing of the Finnish population, a great deal of effort has been put into informing people of the basic elements of good mental health, such as daily routines and maintaining social contacts in other form than face-to-face contacts, and normalizing the feelings of worry. Many NGOs started hotlines, some also multilingually, to serve people suffering from mental health problems due to the COVID-19 situation.

Effect of the COVID-19 pandemic on ethnic relationships has also been raised in public discussion. Particularly following publication of a higher prevalence of COVID-19, among the Somali origin population in the Helsinki area has reportedly increased experiences of blatant discrimination (Kangasluoma & Salomaa 2020).

Conclusions

All things considered, Finland has managed well through the first wave of COVID-19. Containment of the spread of the disease through highly restrictive measures has been effective. Selection of the strategy for dealing with a public threat such as COVID-19 requires balancing between the choice of measures that are highly effective for containment of the threat and the consequences that these bear for the health, economic aspects and the psychosocial wellbeing of the population. THL recently received funding for conducting the Impact of coronavirus epidemic on wellbeing among foreign born population (MigCOVID) Survey that will provide information on the consequences of restrictive measures for the foreign born population in Finland (THL 2020). These findings will contribute to decision-making regarding the uptake of restrictive measures in case of a repetitive public health threat and will guide the reconstructive measures following the COVID-19 pandemic in Finland.

References

Border Guard Organization. (2020). New restrictions on border crossings. Updated April 8th 2020. [referred: 15.7.2020]. Access method: https://www.raja.fi/current_issues/headlines/1/0/new_restrictions_on_border_crossings_79409

Castaneda AE, Cilenti K, Mäki-Opas J, Abdulhamed R, Garoff F (2020). Psyykkinen hyvinvointi. In: Kuusio H, Seppänen A, Jokela S, Somersalo L, Lilja E. Ulkomaalaistaustaisten terveys ja hyvinvointi Suomessa: FinMonik-tutkimus 2018–2019. Publication of THL, Report 1/2020.

Centers for Disease Control and Prevention (CDC). (2020). Weekly Updates by Select Demographic and Geographic Characteristics. National Center for Health Statistics. [referred: 14.7.2020]. Access method: https://www.cdc.gov/nchs/nvss/vsrr/covid_weekly/index.htm#Race_Hispanic

Cuijpers P, Smits N, Donker T, ten Have M, de Graaf R (2009). Screening for mood and anxiety disorders with the five-item, the three-item, and the two-item Mental Health Inventory. Psychiatry Research 168(3), s. 250–255

Eronen A, Hiilamo H, Ilmarinen K, Jokela M, Karjalainen P, Karvonen S, Kivipelto M, Koponen E, Leemann L, Londén P, Saikku P. Socialbarometer (2020). [referred: 16.7.2020]. Access method: https://www.soste.fi/wp-content/uploads/2020/07/SOSBARO2020_EN_final_0307.pdf

Finell, Eerika (2020). Tiedote 3. 2020 Selvitys: Kielivähemmistöjen tiedonsaanti ja kokemukset koronavirusepidemian aikana 23.3 – 20.4.2020. Tampere: Tampereen yliopisto.

Finnish Government. (2020a). Government, in cooperation with the President of the Republic, declares a state of emergency in Finland over coronavirus outbreak. [referred: 13.7.2020]. Access method: https://valtioneuvosto.fi/-/10616/hallitus-totesi-suomen-olevan-poikkeusoloissa-koronavirustilanteen-vuoksi?languageId=en_US

Finnish Government. (2020b). Movement restrictions to Uusimaa - the Government decided on further measures to prevent the spread of the coronavirus epidemic. [referred: 13.7.2020]. Access method: https://valtioneuvosto.fi/-/10616/uudellemaalle-liikkumisrajoituksia-hallitus-paatti-uusista-lisatoimista-koronaepidemian-leviamisen-estamiseksi?languageId=en_US

Finnish Government. (2020c). Use of powers under the Emergency Powers Act to end – state of emergency to be lifted on Tuesday 16 June. [referred: 13.7.2020]. Access method:https://valtioneuvosto.fi/-/10616/valmiuslain-mukaistenztoimivaltuuksien-kaytosta-luovutaan-poikkeusolot-paattyvat-tiistaina-16-kesakuuta?languageId=en_US

Finnish Government. (2020d). [Instructions by the Imam leaders on how to spend Ramadan during the COVID-19 epidemic]. Video material. [referred: 13.7.2020]. Access method: https://twitter.com/valtioneuvosto/status/1260141757947314177

Finnish Immigration Service. 2020a. Only a few asylum applications have been submitted during the coronavirus pandemic. [referred: 16.7.2020]. Access method: https://migri.fi/en/-/koronaviruspandemian-aikana-on-jatetty-vain-vahan-turvapaikkahakemuksia

Finnish Immigration Service. (2020b). Good progress has been made in processing the seasonal work applications. [referred: 16.7.2020]. Access method: https://migri.fi/en/-/kausityohakemusten-kasittely-on-edennyt-pitkalle

Finnish Immigration Service. (2020c). [The quarantine in the Espoo reception centre is over]. [referred: 13.7.2020]. Access method: https://migri.fi/-/espoon-vastaanottokeskuksen-karanteeni-on-paattynyt

Heiskanen R, Saatsi S. (2020). [Thailand demands guaranteed salary and COVID-19 tests for berry workers in Finland, decision on their arrival still pending] The Helsingin Sanomat. [referred: 13.7.2020]. Access method: https://www.hs.fi/kotimaa/art-2000006566773.html

Helsinki City Executive Office. (2020). [Increase in corona virus infections among the Somali origin population] City of Helsinki. [referred: 15.7.2020]. Access method: https://www.hs.fi/kotimaa/art-2000006566773.html

Honkatukia J. [Effects of the pandemic on national economy]. [referred: 5.7.2020]. Access method: https://thl.fi/fi/web/hyvinvoinnin-ja-terveyden-edistamisen-johtaminen/ajankohtaista/koronan-vaikutukset-yhteiskuntaan-ja-palveluihin

Kangasluoma E, Salomaa M. (2020). [Corona virus is spreading among the Somali community, discrimination has become increasingly explicit]. The Helsingin Sanomat. [referred: 15.7.2020]. Access method: https://www.hs.fi/kaupunki/art-2000006479322.html

Koponen P, Rask S, Skogberg N, Castaneda A, Manderbacka K, Suvisaari J, Kuusio H, Laatikainen T, Keskimäri I, Koskinen S. (2016). [Utilization of health services in Finland among persons of foreign origin, In Finnish, English summary available] Suomen Lääkärilehti, 12-13(71), 907-914.

Loula P. (2020). [Nine agricultural workers were diagnosed with COVID-19 in Päijät-Häme – approximately 80 persons in quarantine.] The Helsingin Sanomat. [referred: 15.7.2020]. Access method: https://www.hs.fi/kotimaa/art-2000006569585.html

Ministry of the Interior. (2019). International Migration 2018–2019 –Report for Finland. Ministry of the Interior Publications 2019:32 [referred: 7.7.2020]. Access method: http://urn.fi/URN:ISBN:978-952-324-303-3.

Ministry of Justice. (2003). Emergency Powers Act. [referred: 7.7.2020]. Access method: https://www.finlex.fi/fi/laki/kaannokset/1991/en19911080_20030696.pdf

Norwegian Institute of Public Health. (2020). Weekly reports for coronavirus and COVID-19. [referred: 7.7.2020]. Access method: https://www.fhi.no/contentassets/8a971e7b0a3c4a06bdbf381ab52e6157/2020.07.08-ukerapport-uke-27-covid-19-versjon-2.pdf

Official Statistics of Finland (OSF). (2020a). Maahanmuuttajat väestössä [*Immigrants in the population*, e-publication]. Helsinki: Statistics Finland [referred: 7.7.2020]. Access method: http://www.stat.fi/tup/maahanmuutto/maahanmuuttajat-vaestossa.html#tab1485503695201_2

Official Statistics of Finland (OSF). (2020b). Population structure [e-publication]. ISSN=1797-5395. Annual Review 2019. Helsinki: Statistics Finland [referred: 7.7.2020]. Access method: http://www.stat.fi/til/vaerak/2019/02/vaerak_2019_02_2020-05-29_tie_001_en.html

Onali A. (2020). [Finland prohibits back-and-forth traveling of Estonian workers]. The Helsingin Sanomat. [referred: 7.7.2020]. Access method: https://www.hs.fi/kaupunki/art-2000006446347.html

Public Health Agency of Sweden. (2020). [Demographic description of COVID-19 insidence in Sweden between March 13th and May 7th]. [referred: 7.7.2020]. Access method: http://www.folkhalsomyndigheten.se/publiceratmaterial/publikationsarkiv/c/demografisk-beskrivning-av-bekraftade-covid-19-fall-i-sverige-13-mars-7-maj-2020/

Parhiala K, Jormanainen V. (2020). [Services and benefits]. Finnish Institute for Health and Welfare [referred: 7.7.2020]. Access method: https://thl.fi/fi/web/hyvinvoinnin-ja-terveyden-edistamisen-johtaminen/ajankohtaista/koronan-vaikutukset-yhteiskuntaan-ja-palveluihin

Platt L, Warwick R. (2020). Are some ethnic groups more vulnerable to COVID-19 than others? Institute for Fiscal Studies. [referred: 15.7.2020]. Access: file:///C:/Users/nsoz/AppData/Local/Temp/Are-some-ethnic-groups-more-vulnerable-to%20COVID-19-than-others-V2-IFS-Briefing-Note.pdf

Rask S, Suvisaari J, Koskinen S, Koponen P, Mölsä M, Lehtisalo R, Schubert C, Pakaslahti A, Castaneda AE (2016c). The ethnic gap in mental health: a population-based study of Russian, Somali and Kurdish origin migrants in Finland. Scandinavian Journal of Public Health 44(3), s. 281–290.

Ruokakangas P. [Will traveling for work across the border from Lapland end?] Yle News 30.3.2020. [referred: 15.7.2020]. Access method: https://yle.fi/uutiset/3-11282172

Saukkonen P. 2020. [Coronavirus and international mobility]. Kvartti. [referred: 15.7.2020]. Access: https://www.kvartti.fi/fi/blogit/koronavirus-ja-kansainvalinen-muuttoliike

Skogberg N, Adam A, Kinnunen T, Castaneda A. (2018). Overweight and Obesity among Russian, Somali, and Kurdish Origin Populations in Finland. Finnish Yearbook of Population Research,53:73-87.

Skogberg N, Laatikainen T, Koskinen S, Vartiainen E, Jula A, Leiviskä J, Härkänen T, Koponen P. (2016). Cardiovascular risk factors among Russian, Somali and Kurdish migrants in comparison with the general Finnish population. Eurn J Public Health, 26(4), 667-73.

Sutela H. (2015). Ulkomaalaistaustaiset työelämässä [e-publication]. Helsinki: Statistics

Finland [Multilingual information on the corona virus][referred: 7.7.2020]. Access method: https://www.stat.fi/tup/maahanmuutto/art_2015-12-17_003.html

THL (Finnish Institute for Health and Welfare) (2020). Impact of coronavirus epidemic on wellbeing among foreign born population (MigCOVID) Survey. [referred: 17.7.2020]. Access method: thl.fi/en/migcovid.

THL (Finnish Institute for Health and Welfare) (2020a). [Overview of the corona virus situation in Finland]. [referred: 16.7.2020]. Access method: https://thl.fi/fi/web/infektiotaudit-ja-rokotukset/ajankohtaista/ajankohtaista-koronaviruksesta-covid-19/tilannekatsaus-koronaviruksesta

THL (Finnish Institute for Health and Welfare) (2020b). [Several clusters of COVID-19 found at construction cites]. [referred: 5.7.2020]. Access method: https://thl.fi/fi/-/rakennustyomailla-todettu-useita-tautirypaita-suomessa-koronaepidemian-torjuntaa-tehostettava-tyomailla

THL (Finnish Institute for Health and Welfare) (2020c). [Multilingual information on the corona virus]. [referred: 13.7.2020]. Access method: https://thl.fi/fi/web/infektiotaudit-ja-rokotukset/ajankohtaista/ajankohtaista-koronaviruksesta-covid-19/materiaalipankki-koronaviruksesta/koronatietoa-eri-kielilla

THL (Finnish Institute for Health and Welfare) (2020d). [Spend Ramadan safely with your family]. Finnish National Intitute for Health and Welfare. [referred 13.7.2020]. Access method: https://twitter.com/THLorg/status/12536530617609 25696

Yle News. (2020). Russian tourists eager to book holidays in Finland despite border closure. [referred 13.7.2020]. Access method: https://yle.fi/uutiset/osasto/news/russian_   tourists_eager_to_book_holidays_in_finland_despite_border_closure/11430543.

CHAPTER 13

REMITTANCES FROM MEXICAN MIGRANTS IN THE UNITED STATES DURING COVID-19

Rodolfo García Zamora and Selene Gaspar Olvera

According to the World Bank, remittances around the world will fall about 20% as a result of the economic crisis created by the COVID-19 pandemic and associated lockdowns. The projected drop, which will be the sharpest fall in recent history, is largely due to the collapse of migrant workers' wages and employment—workers who are often more vulnerable to the loss of jobs and wages during economic crises in the countries that host them. In light of these predictions, remittances will fall 19.7%, dropping to US$445 billion dollars compared to US$554 billion dollars the previous year. The World Bank predicts that the biggest drops will be in Europe and Central Asia (27.5%), followed by Sub-Saharan Africa (23.1%), South Asia (22.1%), the Middle East and North Africa (19.6%), Latin America and the Caribbean (19.3%) and East Asia and the Pacific (13%). Even when taking this trend into account, the institution considers that remittances will continue to be a very important source of financing for recipient countries compared to direct foreign investment, which it estimates will fall by more than 35% in 2020. This maintains the trend seen in recent years of larger amounts of remittances than direct foreign investment (World Bank, 2020).

For the World Bank, the outlook for remittances remains as uncertain as the impact of COVID-19 on prospects for global growth and the measures implemented to restrict the spread of the virus. In the past, remittances have been countercyclical: workers send more money home when their home countries are experiencing crisis and hardship. This time, however, the pandemic has affected every country in the world, creating additional uncertainties. In the face of this scenario, the Bank points out that effective social protection systems are crucial to protect poor and vulnerable populations during the present crisis, both in developing countries and advanced economies.

Remittances sent by Mexican migrants living in the United States during the past five decades have also followed the global growth trend—despite the labour, economic and immigration policy obstacles that Mexicans encounter in the country, they continue to send family and collective remittances to their home communities at increasing levels. While the number of Mexican migrants has multiplied 1.8 times since 1995, from 6.96 million to 12.26 million in 2018, international remittances have increased 9.2 times, rising from US$3.673 to US$33.677 billion in the same observation period (Figure 13.1). Despite the high unemployment rates experienced by Mexican immigrants during the United States' 2007-2009 economic recession, their remittances reached a level of over US$21 billion dollars. As the recession began to subside, remittance levels rose as a result of increasing employment rates for Mexicans. During economic contractions, the unemployment rate among Mexican migrants' increases, then decreases at the slightest indication of economic recovery. The flow of remittances, therefore increases (Delgado and Gaspar, 2018; García and Gaspar, 2019). Migrant exports become the most profitable source of foreign currency in the country; yet despite their importance, migrants are not a priority for the current government, such that a reduction of Program resources and an elimination of sources of support is what they receive in return (García, Gaspar and Del Valle, 2019).

Figure 13.1. GDP growth rate in the United States, 2006-2019 and international remittance levels in Mexico, 2006-2019

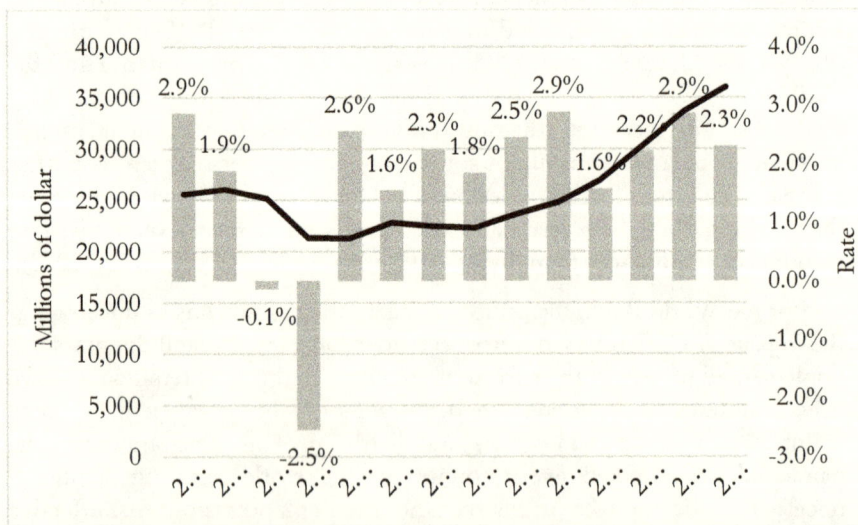

Source: SIMDE-UAZ. Prepared by the authors with Bank of Mexico data.

Data from the World Bank shows that Mexico occupies the third position in a ranking of highest remittance levels (US$33.677 billion according to data from the Bank of Mexico), India coming first with US$78.609 billion, and China in second position (US$67.414 billion). The indicator for remittances as a percentage of GDP highlights the importance of remittances from migrants for the Mexican economy; here it places first with 3.0%, India second (2.9%) and China has a rate of 0.5%.

According to the United Nations (2019), family remittances have a direct impact on the lives of one billion people, this being three times more than Official Development Assistance and exceeding Foreign Direct Investment. Collective remittances are monetary funds or donations that migrant organizations or clubs send, mainly to their communities of origin, as a way to sponsor community projects.

Migrants' individual and collective remittances have multiplier effects, given that they strengthen the economy by increasing demand for goods and services. Both types of remittances have positive effects on the development of human capital, since in both cases resources are allocated for education; children from migrant households achieve between 0.7 and 1.6 more years of education than children from non-migrant households (OIM, 51, citing Duryea *et al.*, 2005). In terms of their impact on health, it has been found that for Mexican households, receiving remittances is a significant economic determinant of spending money on medical care, and also reduces child mortality. As such, a decrease in remittances can affect the households that receive them in a variety of ways (Amuedo and Pozo, 2009; López Córdoba, 2004; Duryea *et al.*, 2005 cited in García and Pérez, 2008).

In 2018, more than 1.6 million households in Mexico received international remittances; for households that receive them they represent 56.1% of transfers, in rural areas for non-poor households they represent 59.2%, and for households in poverty, 55.1%. It is worth mentioning that for households with remittances, transfers represent 49.8% of their total monetary income. In Mexico's agriculture sector, investment in livestock increases (IOM, citing Taylor, 1992). Furthermore, a recent study carried out in Chiapas finds that adoption of modern technologies is highest in the group of producers who receive remittances—this translates to higher performance, demonstrating the contribution remittances make towards productivity (Tuirán, Ramírez, Damián, Juárez and Estrella, 2015).

Remittances operate as one of the most important and dynamic sources of foreign exchange (Delgado and Gaspar, 2018). They reduce negative impacts on other sources of foreign exchange during economic contractions and offer temporary relief in poverty reduction, yet they are vulnerable to its fluctuations (García and Gaspar, 2019). Aragonés and Salgado (2015) point out that while remittances play an important role in terms of Mexico's macroeconomic stability, promoting the country's development necessitates a radical transformation of the conditions that have forced men and women to emigrate.

Since the beginning of the 21st century, with the growth of migration and remittances in the world—especially in Latin America and the Caribbean—there has been broad debate regarding the importance and impacts of remittances on migrants' countries and communities of origin, and whether this flow should be seen as fostering development or as transfers that help improve the living conditions and well-being of the receiving families. García Zamora (2006) points out that international migration and remittances can mitigate marginalization and poverty, however, by themselves they cannot overcome poverty or generate economic development in a country. Remittances provide temporary relief for family poverty, but rarely offer a permanent path to financial security (Orozco, 2005). Thus, although this monetary resource has been found to reduce family poverty, it also creates dependency and vulnerability when remittances are reduced or no longer received (Delgado and Gaspar 2018), and the State becomes the most important institution in overcoming it (Canales Cerón, 2008).

Alejandro Canales points out that in order to understand the economic and social significance of remittances in today's world, it is essential to locate international migration in the context of structural changes to the world economy under globalization. In this process, various mechanisms of social inclusion and exclusion are activated, which—through the precariousness of employment and other forms of social segregation—have given rise to further patterns of transnational social polarization and differentiation. Remittances are generated by precarious and vulnerable workers living in destination countries who send transfers to their families living in conditions of poverty and social marginalization. Within this context, it is shown that remittances are mainly destined for family consumption and help to maintain a minimum of well-being, and that they are insufficient to drive a meaningful process of social mobility and economic development in communities of origin (García Zamora, 2009).

The amount of family remittances sent by Mexican migrants in the United States before the 2007-2009 Great Recession saw an increasing trend, as occurred worldwide, while during the recession, the amount of remittances decreased more in Mexico as compared to the global trend. After variations during the first few years after the recession, remittances recovered again and reached unprecedented levels, with a historic level in 2017 of US\$30.261 billion. This recovery may have been due to an increase in employment, rather than an increase in Mexican emigration, which has remained close to 12 million.

Data from the United Nations (UN, 2017) shows that the United States remains the primary destination for international migrants and Mexican immigration, despite the stock stagnation that it has experienced for ten years, the reduction in emigration flows and the increase in return migration to

Mexico; Mexicans are the largest group of immigrants in the United States, and Mexico is the nation with the most migration between two countries (Ávila and Gaspar, 2018). In 2017, Mexican immigrants in the United States totaled 12.2 million, a population historically constituted by work-focused emigration at a reproductive age—circumstances which have resulted in a population of 13.6 million Americans with at least one parent born in Mexico, and 11.8 million Americans who identify themselves as being of Mexican descent. This situation explains why 94.8% of the 30.29 billion dollars of remittances that Mexico received in 2017 came from the United States. In fact, our country ranks second in having the largest number of inhabitants outside its territory, and occupies the fourth position in biggest remittance recipients after India, China and the Philippines.

Figure 13.2. World and Mexico. Family remittances 1994-2017

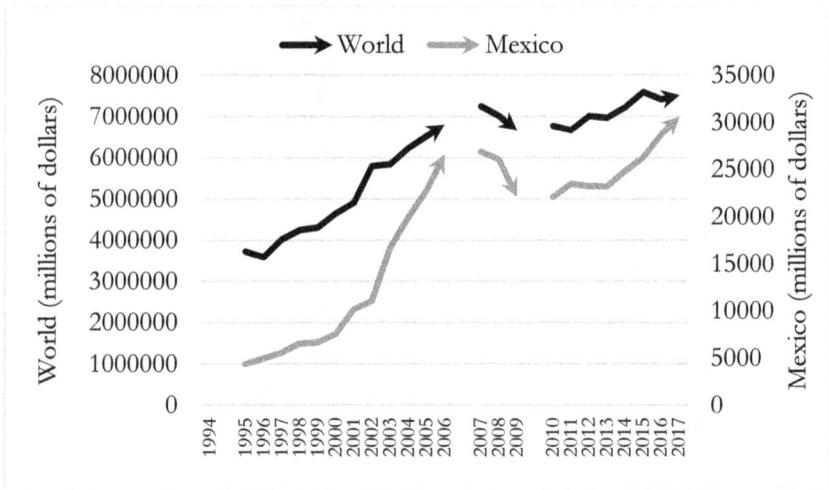

Source: SIMDE-UAZ. Prepared by the authors with World Bank data.

Mexicans' family remittances show exponential growth from 1994 to 2007. After 2007, given changes in the American economy and immigration policy, Mexican migration to the United States saw important changes in stock growth and the emigration flows to the country. These changes were intensified with the economic crisis that began in late 2007, which affected employment of Mexicans and remittances sent to Mexico. Figures 13.2 to 13.4 shows the effects of the 2007-2009 economic contraction on Mexican immigrants' employment in the United States and on remittances sent to Mexico; the effects are notable for both items in 2009.

According to the Bureau of Labor Statistics, during the Great Recession of 2007-2009 the economy contracted sharply and nearly 8.7 million jobs were lost. Of these, 3.2 million were jobs linked to consumer demand, an area which experienced the steepest decline since World War II as a result of the drop in household spending. During the recession, Mexican migrants lost 232,000 jobs in 2008 and 353,000 in 2009—the year in which the Mexican unemployment rate reached its highest level at 13.3%, though this recovered quickly and in 2016 it saw the same levels as before the recession (5.1%). In this context, remittances decreased more intensely; while the decrease in employment was 5.0% in 2009, for remittances it was 15.2% (US$3.996 billion). After 2010, unemployment of Mexicans fell and remittances began their recovery.

Figure 13.3. Mexican immigrants in the United States and family remittances

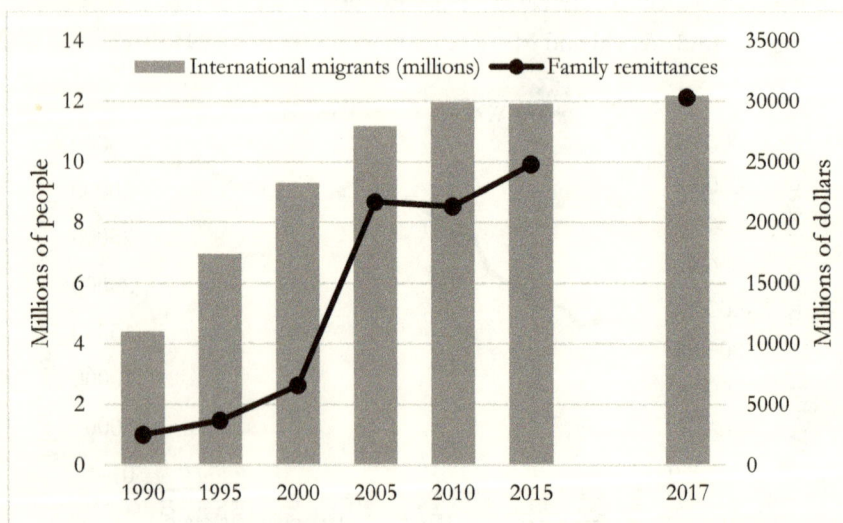

Source: SIMDE-UAZ. Prepared by the authors based on U.S. Census Bureau data for selected years, and data from the Bank of Mexico.

In 2020, the impact of COVID-19 on the American economy, with the expected 5.9% contraction of the GDP and 36 million unemployed in May, implies the most severe economic crisis since the Great Depression of 1929. Serious impacts have been observed on unemployment in general and for Mexican migrants in particular, who saw 17.5% unemployment at the end of April, a number which translates to 1.2 million people. This situation affects just over 1.5 million households which have at least one Mexican among its members; in these households there are at least 2.1 million people unemployed. In this scenario, 6.8 million people—Mexican immigrants and people born in the United States who belong to such households—see reduced income and less economic stability which they require to meet their basic daily needs. These circumstances may lead to an increased flow of

Mexican migrants returning to Mexico, above the levels of recent years which are between 100,000 and 130,000 returnees. The return numbers could become equivalent to or greater than those seen during the 2007-2009 Great Recession, when 300,000 people returned to Mexico and unemployment was at 13.3%. This potentially higher number of returnees finds Mexico with its own problems, dealing with the impacts of the dual pandemics (health and economic) and having an expected 6.6% contraction of the GDP and 1.5 million workers unemployed, added to the 7 million people who are chronically unemployed. In the Mexican case, effects on unemployment and the GDP will depend on the duration of the dual pandemics, the response capacity of the health sector, and results of the Mexican government's economic recovery policy (García and Olvera, 2020b).

Figure 13.4. Absolute increase in Mexican immigrants' employment in the United States and family remittances that Mexico received, 2001-2017

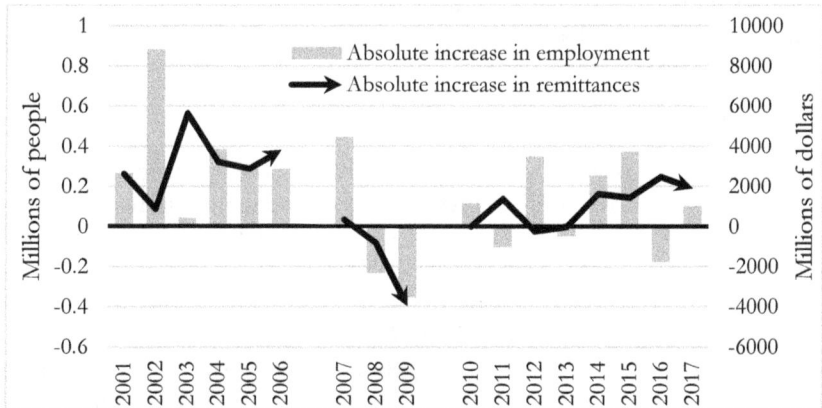

Source: SIMDE-UAZ. Prepared by the authors based on the U.S. Census Bureau Current Population Survey (CPS-ASEC) for selected years, and data from the Bank of Mexico.

In Mexico, in 2019 remittances sent from the United States reached their highest level in history at US$36.046 billion, a growth of 7% and higher than flows of direct foreign investment and oil exports (El Financiero, February 4, 2020). Paradoxically, in March of 2020, when the health and economic impacts of COVID-19 were growing in the United States and Mexico, remittances received in Mexico grew surprisingly and reached a historical level of US$4.016 billion—35.8% more than in March 2019, and due to a higher number of shipments and more operations (Forbes México, May 4). Viri Ríos argues that the historical increase in remittances means that migrants are rescuing Mexico and López Obrador. Remittances are a lifeline for millions of Mexican families, and could also be a salve for the president's popularity (The New York Times, May 19, 2020). However, in the month of April, remittances sent to Mexico suffered a 28.5% drop compared to the previous month, measuring at US$2.861 billion. This is the largest monthly drop in remittances since November 2008. The reduction essentially means an amount of US$329 compared to US$377 the previous month; the number of transfers was similar to that of the previous year.

For the Banorte Financial Group, factors that may contribute to a fall in the flow of remittances include employment in the United States and restrictions on mobility along the northern border. Regarding the first factor, they point out that Mexican migrants lost almost 3 million jobs: "natives," children of Mexican parents born in the United States, lost 1.8 million; "non-native citizens" lost 202,000; and "non-citizens," which includes undocumented workers, lost 911,000 jobs. The second factor, introduced with the presidential initiative of March 21 aimed at restricting international mobility, has further reduced the migratory flow between the two countries (Rodríguez and Guzmán 2020, June 1, 2020). The Center for Latin American Monetary Studies estimates that in April Mexican migrants in the United States lost 1,973,897 jobs (representing one in four Mexicans in the country), resulting in an unemployment rate of 17% (La Jornada, June 3, 2020).

Conclusion

Over the past 30 years, remittances received in Mexico from migrants in the United States have been of great macroeconomic importance, in recent years exceeding direct foreign investment and income from oil exports, and benefiting more than 1.6 million households in an informal welfare system where those who have migrated help their families in their home communities. Those that benefit from such transfers are simultaneously very vulnerable to their reduction or suspension. The correlation between an increase of 17% in unemployment of Mexican migrants in the United States and a drop of 28% in remittances sent in April is clear, affecting their families' well-being while increasing uncertainty for the future. Recuperating the amount of remittances sent to Mexico will depend on the effectiveness of policies aimed at economic recovery in the United States, particularly in sectors with the biggest presence of Mexican migrants, such as food, lodging, recreation, industry, commerce, services and construction.

References

Amuedo-Dorantes, C. and S. Pozo (2009). New evidence on the role of remittances on health care expenditures by Mexican households, IZA Discussion Papers, No. 4617, Institute for the Study of Labor (IZA), Bonn. https://www.econstor.eu/bitstream/10419/36035/1/617543798.pdf

Aragonés, C., A. María and U. S. Nieto (2015). La migración laboral México-Estados Unidos a veinte años del Tratado de Libre Comercio de América del Norte. Revista Mexicana de Ciencias Políticas y Sociales. UNAM. Nueva Época, Year LX, no. 224, pp. 279-314. http://www.revistas.unam.mx/index.php/rmcpys/article/view/49218/44960

Banco Mundial (2020). El Banco Mundial prevé la mayor caída de remesas de la historia reciente. April 22.

Canales, C. (2008). Remesas y desarrollo. Una relación en busca de teoría, inédito.

Canales, Al. and S. Meza (2016). Fin del colapso y nuevo escenario migratorio México-Estados Unidos. Migración y Desarrollo No. 27 Second semester 2016. http://www.scielo.org.mx/pdf/myd/v14n27/1870-7599-myd-14-27-00065.pdf

Córdova, K. (2009). Collective Remittances in Mexico: Their Effect on the Labor Market for Males. https://pdfs.semanticscholar.org/5897/ef3d7f6fa7d3f8307 c78a1e5b6e262b9c622.pdf

Delgado, W. R. and S. G. Olvera (2018). Confrontando el discurso dominante: Las remesas bajo el prisma de la experiencia mexicana. REMHU, Rev. Interdiscip. Mobil. Hum., Brasília, v. 26, n. 52, Apr. 2018, p. 243-263 http://www.scielo.br/pdf/remhu/v26n52/2237-9843-remhu-26-52-243.pdf

El Financiero (2020). "Ingreso récord de remesas en 2019", February 4. https://www.elfinanciero.com.mx/nacional/remesas-familiares-crecen-7-04-y-alcanzan-cifra-record-durante-el-2019

Forbes México (2020). "Remesas a México sorprenden con récord en marzo pese a coronoavirus", May 4. https://www.forbes.com.mx/economia-remesas-mexico-marzo-record-pese-coronavirus/

García Zamora, R. (2006). "Migración internacional y desarrollo: Los proyectos de los Clubes zacatecanos en California", in Migraciones en América Latina. Un Continente en movimiento. Iberoamericana-Vervuet, Madrid.

García Zamora, R. (2009). Desarrollo económico y migración internacional: los desafíos de las políticas públicas en México. Universidad Autónoma de Zacatecas

García Zamora, R. and S.G. Olvera (2019). Crisis migratoria y de fronteras bajo la jaula neoliberal en México. Brújula Ciudadana 109. https://www. revistabrujula.org/copia-de-b109-heredia

García Zamora, R. and S.G. Olvera (2019). La gran recesión 2007-2009 e impacto en las remesas en México. Vol. 11 (No. 31) September- December 2018, http://www. olafinanciera.unam.mx/new_web/31/pdfs/PDF31/GarciaGasparOlaFin31.pdf

García Zamora, R. and S.G. Olvera (2020). El COVID-19, los inmigrantes mexicanos en Estados Unidos y la migración de retorno a México. Impactos en el empleo y los hogares (Unpublished).

García Zamora, R., S. G. Olvera and R. E. del Valle Martínez (2019). "Crisis rural, violencias crecientes y desplome migratorio: la reproducción de la sociedad rural en su encrucijada en la 4 Transformación". Coloquio XLI de Antropología e historia regionales. Extraños en su tierra. Sociedades rurales en tiempos del neoliberalismo: Escenarios en Transición del 2 al 4 de octubre 2019. El colegio de Michoacán.

García Zamora, R. (2019). México. La Nación desafiada. Análisis y propuesta ante la migración y la falta de desarrollo en México. Miguel Ángel Porrúa-Universidad Autónoma de Zacatecas. México, Zacatecas.

García Zamora, R. and O. P. Veyna (2008). Migración internacional, organizaciones de migrantes y desarrollo local en El Salvador, Michoacán y Zacatecas. Pp.189-211. In Desarrollo Económico y Migración Internacional: Los desafíos de las políticas públicas en México. Rodolfo García Zamora. Colección Ángel Migrante. http://ricaxcan.uaz.edu.mx/jspui/bitstream/20.500.11845/40/1/Migra%20Angel.p df

García Zamora, R. (2008). Migración internacional y desarrollo en América Latina y el Caribe: del mito a la realidad. Pp.13-36. In Desarrollo Económico y Migración Internacional: Los desafíos de las políticas públicas en México. Rodolfo García Zamora. Colección Ángel Migrante. http://ricaxcan.uaz.edu.mx/jspui/bitstream/ 20.500.11845/40/1/Migra%20Angel.pdf

Naciones Unidas (2019). International Day of Family Remittances, June 16.

https://www.un.org/en/observances/remittances-day

Rodríguez, S. and K. Guzmán (2020). "Envío de remesas a México cae 28.5%" in Milenio, June 1. https://www.milenio.com/negocios/remesas-mexico-caen-28-5-abril-2020-banxico

Rodríguez, I. (2020). "Perdieron empleo en abril uno de cada cuatro mexicanos en Estados Unidos. Causa baja en las remesas. CEMLA", La Jornada, June 3. https://www.jornada.com.mx/2020/06/03/economia/021n1eco

The New York Times (2020) "Los migrantes rescatan a México y a López Obrador", May 19. https://www.nytimes.com/es/2020/05/19/espanol/opinion/remesas-mexico.html

Tuirán-Altamirano, T., Ramírez-Valverde, B., Damián-Huato, M. Á., Juárez-Sánchez, J.P., and Estrella-Chulím, N. (2015). Uso de remesas para la adquisición de tecnología agrícola en maíz en San José Chiapas, Puebla, México. Nova scientia, 7(14), 674-693. http://www.scielo.org.mx/scielo.php?script=sci_arttext&pid=S2007-07052015000200674&lng=es&tlng=es.

CHAPTER 14

THE COVID-19, MIGRATION AND LIVELIHOOD IN INDIA: CHALLENGES AND POLICY ISSUES

R.B. Bhagat, Reshmi R.S., Harihar Sahoo, Archana K. Roy, Dipti Govil

Introduction

The epidemics of the past was hardly concerned with migration and livelihood during the colonial India, although major Indian cities like Kolkata (Calcutta), Mumbai (Bombay), Chennai (Madras) and many other urban places hugely suffered from influenza, smallpox, plague, malaria and cholera (Davis, 1951; Banthia and Dyson, 1999; Hill, 2011). Mumbai experienced a deadly plague in 1896 and also an influenza in 1918. Hill observed that the epidemic of influenza arrived in Mumbai in September 1918 which swept through north and east India. He found that excess mortality due to influenza was negatively related with out-migration at district-level analysis, but offered no explanation (Hill, 2011). Compared to epidemics, famine was seen not only causing mortality but also migration in the past (Maharatna, 2014). In 1994, a major epidemic of plague broke out in western India with epicentre in Surat. There was a huge exodus of migrant population from the industrial city of Surat.

When migrants flee from the city, they not only lose their livelihood but they may carry the infections to their native places (BBC, 2020). In the period of epidemic of HIV/AIDS which broke during the 1980s in various parts of the world, migrants were greatly stigmatized as a carrier of the disease and considered to be a population at risk. This has obliterated the great contribution of migrants in economic growth, innovation, skill development and entrepreneurship in building cities and the nation. On the other hand, policies and programmes of urban development and planning in India hardly launched any specific programmes for the migrants as they were not considered as a part of the urban community. Failure to recognize migrants as a stakeholder in urban development is one of the biggest mistakes in achieving urban sustainability and realizing the goals of sustainable development in India. It is to be realized that migrants are not a victimizer, nor a victim, but they are vulnerable. They are engaged in many 3D jobs (dirty, dangerous and demeaning) which the so-called urban natives hate to do. Access to social security programmes, access to health care and other entitlements are grossly denied to many of these migrant workers due to lack of their inclusion in urban society. Several of them also lose their political rights as being away at the time of election from their home constituency and are not able to vote.

Migrants suffer from the double burden of being poor and migrants. Many programmes meant for the poor do not reach them due to lack of identity and residential proofs. The lack of fulfilment of the economic, social and political rights of migrants is a serious issue even though they are formal citizens, and their substantive citizenship rights are not fulfilled. The Working Group on Migration (2017) set up by the Ministry of Housing and Urban Poverty Alleviation has examined the plight of the migrant workers in the country and submitted its report to Central Government in 2017. However, action on the report is still awaited. In the meantime, the sudden eruption of migration crisis resulting from the outbreak of COVID-19 again reminds us the urgency of the matter. This paper presents how our understanding of migration and livelihood could be helpful in designing a mitigating strategy of the economic and social impact of COVID-19.

Migration and Livelihood

Migration is a livelihood strategy adopted by millions of people in India. Most of the migration for work and employment is directed towards urban centres. About half of the urban population are migrants and one-fifth of them are inter-state migrants (See Figure 14.1). Rural to urban migrants are mainly concentrated in 53 million-plus urban agglomerations (with one million and more) that comprises 140 million out of 377 million urban population of the country equivalent to 43 per cent of total urban population as per 2011 Census. Out of 53 million-plus cities, eight of them are mega-cities with a population of 5 million and more. These eight cities reported about 55 per cent COVID cases of India, although they constitute only 7 per cent of India's population. The relevant information on these eight cities has been provided in Table 14.1.

As on 8th June 2020, the respective districts of eight mega cities reported more than half of the corona virus positive cases.[1] The incidence of COVID 19 shows that these metropolitan areas are the centres from where the disease has been spreading to the near as well as far off places. Migrant workers constitute backbone of Indian economy. Out of 482 million workers in India about 194 millions are permanent and semi-permanent migrant workers (Figure 14.2).

---

[1] https://www.covid19india.org/

Figure 14.1. Migration Intensity and Share of Inter-State Migrants in Rural and Urban Areas, India, 2011

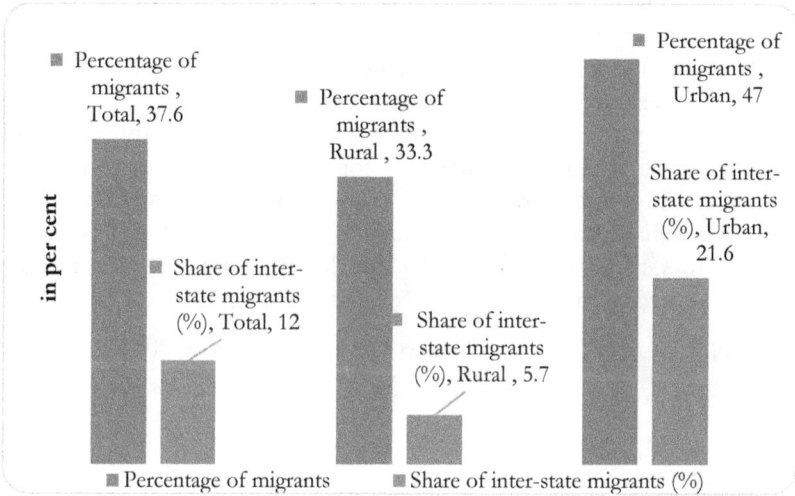

Source: D2 Migration Table, Census of India 2011

Table 14.1. Migration Intensity, Share of Inter-Sate Migrants, India, 2011and Covid-19 Cases in Mega Cities, 2020`

Urban Agglomeration (UA)	Population (2011)	Percentage of migrants to total population	% Share of inter-state migrants to total migrants	Number of COVID cases in the respective districts as on 10th June 2020 (Total Cases in India 279,721)
Delhi	16349831	43.1	87.8	31309
Greater Mumbai	18394912	54.9	46	65163*
Kolkata	14057911	40.8	18.2	3018
Chennai	8653521	51	11.8	25937
Bruhat Banglore	8520435	52.3	35.1	564
Hyderabad	7677018	64.3	7.1	2371
Ahmedabad	6357693	48.7	24.1	14962
Pune	5057709	64.8	22.3	10073
Urban India	**377106125**	**47.0**	**21.6**	Share of Covid19 cases in these metro cities to total cases of India is 55 %

Source: D3 (Appendix) Migration Table, Census of India 2011;
https://www.covid19india.org/ accessed on 10th June, 2020). Note : * indicates total cases in Greater Mumbai Urban agglomeration, ie, Mumbai and Thane districts.

In addition, there are about 15 million short-term migrant workers of temporary and circulatory nature. The inter-state share in labour migration is about one-third for permanent/semi-permanent migration and about two-fifth for short-term temporary and circulatory migration. In general, in-migration rates were high in high-income states such as Delhi, Goa, Haryana, Punjab, Maharashtra, Gujarat and Karnataka, whereas low-income states such as Bihar, Uttar Pradesh, Jharkhand, Rajasthan and Odisha reported relatively higher rates of out-migration (Figure 14.3). Some of the in-migrating states such as Maharashtra, Gujarat and Delhi are badly affected by the incidence of COVID-19. There are conspicuous corridors of migration flows within the country – Bihar to Delhi, Bihar to Haryana and Punjab, Uttar Pradesh to Maharashtra, Odisha to Gujarat, Odisha to Andhra Pradesh and Rajasthan to Gujarat (Bhagat and Keshri 2020). The inter-state migration flow is presented in Figure 14.4.

Figure 14.2. Stock of Migrant Workers (in million), India, 2011

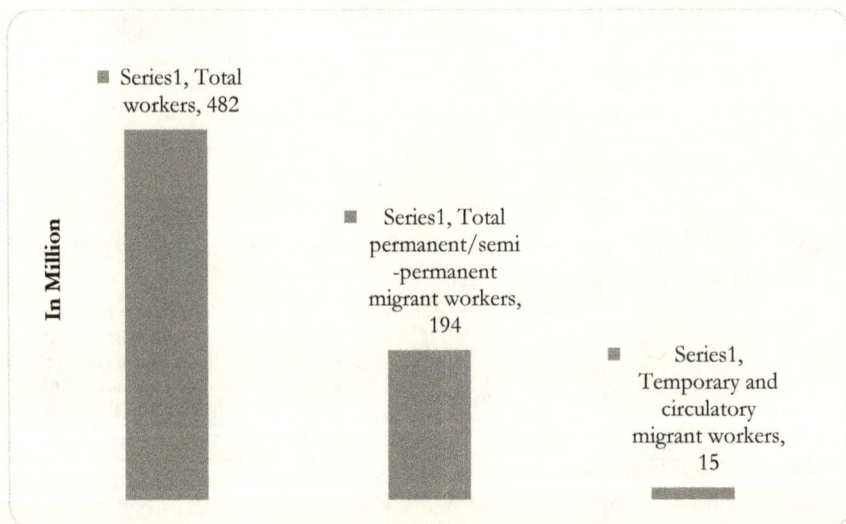

Note: Total workers and total permanent/semi-permanent migrant workers are based on B1 Economic Table and D6 Migration Table of Census of India 2011. It includes both main and marginal workers. Temporary and circulatory migration is the short-term migration based on NSS 64th Round. Based on the rate of NSS 64th Round for the year 2007-08 it is projected for the census year 2011 (see also Keshri and Bhagat 2012).

When workers do not get any option for livelihood and employment and there is an expectation of economic improvement in the place of origin, labour migration takes place (Lall, Selod and Shalizi, 2006). In many cases, they work and stay in an urban area for a long time while in other cases, short term or temporary migration become livelihood strategies of the rural poor. The National Commission for Enterprises in the Unorganised Sector (NCEUS) reports around 92 per cent of India's workforce with informal employment are substantially drawn from migrant labour (NCEUS, 2007). About 30 per cent of migrant workers are working as casual workers, are therefore quite vulnerable to the vagaries of the labour market and lack social protection. Only 35 per cent of migrant workers are employed as regular/salaried workers (NSSO, 2010).

Figure 14.3. State-wise Net Migration Rates (NMR %) (0-4 years of migration duration), 2011

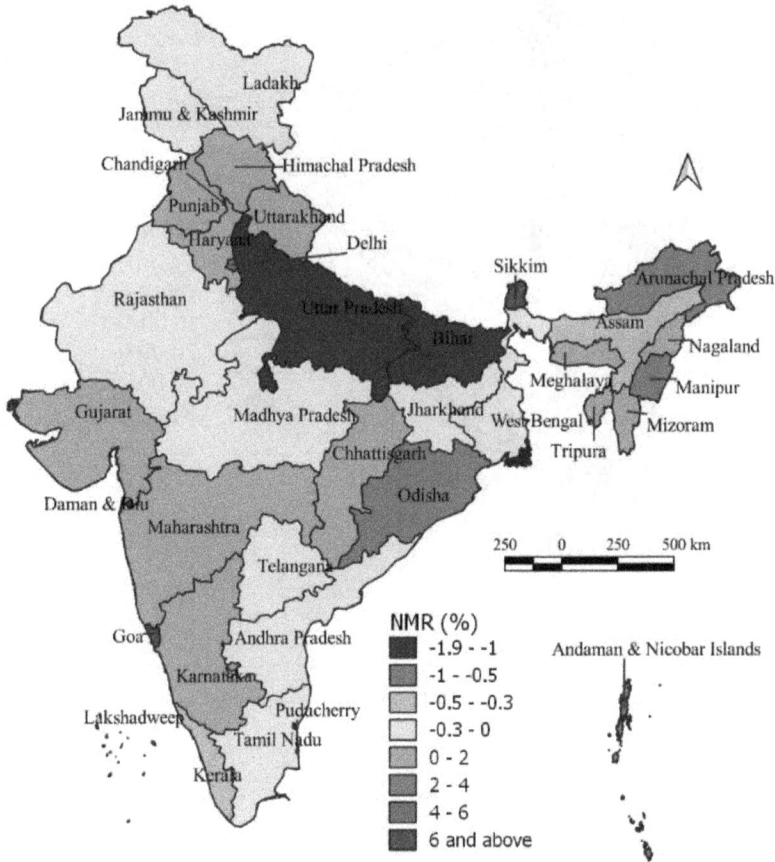

Source: Census of India 2011, D-2 Migration Table (www.censusindia.gov.in).

Figure 14.4. Net Migration Flows between States, duration 0-4 years, 2011

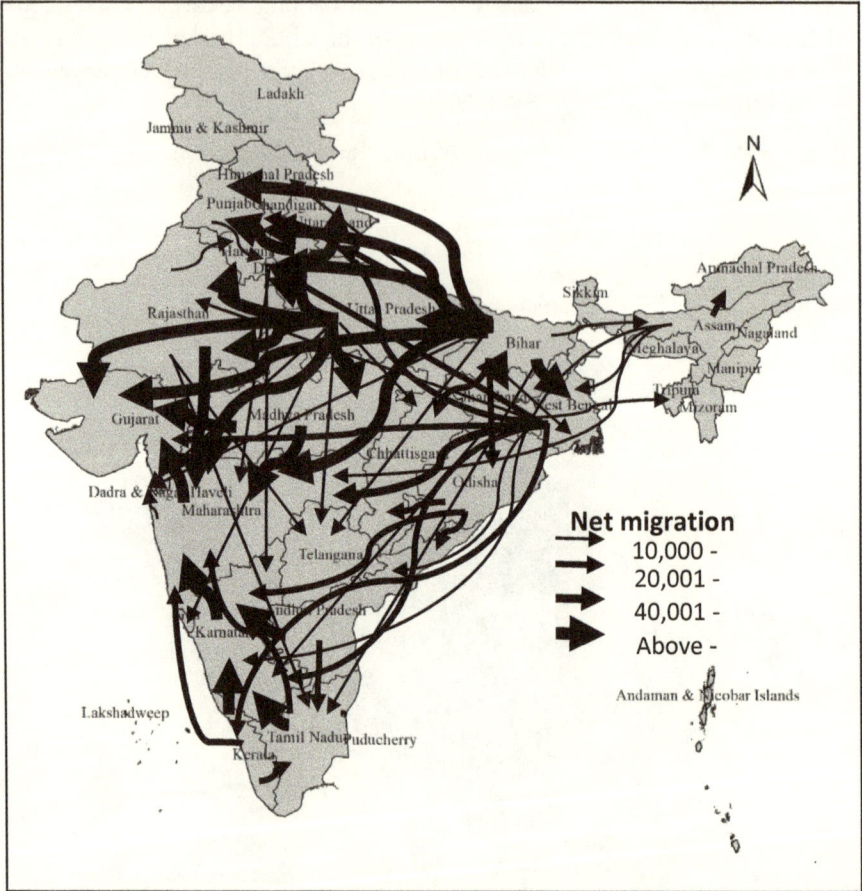

Source: Calculated from Census of India 2011, D-2 Migration Table
(www.censusindia.gov.in).

Impact of COVID-19 on Migrant Workers

The spread of Coronavirus from the epicentre of Wuhan in China to worldwide is attributed to migration and mobility of people. The medical professionals largely believe that the control of this infectious disease is possible through immobility and confinement like lockdown and social distancing. Moreover, in a globalised world, the lockdown is likely to bring an unprecedented breakdown of our economic and social system. Migrants are most vulnerable to urban disasters and epidemics. The first case of COVID-19 surfaced in India on January 30, 2020, and following the outbreak the lockdown in the entire country was announced on 24th March for a period of 21days. Borders were sealed, transportation was ceased, factories, shops, restaurants and all type of the economic activities were shut, barring only the essential services. This proved to be a nightmare for hundreds of thousands of migrant workers, who lost their livelihoods overnight and became homeless. The immediate challenges faced by these migrant workers were related to food, shelter, loss of wages, fear of getting infected and anxiety. As a result, thousands of them started fleeing from various cities to their native places. Many migrants lost their lives either due to hardship on the way to their destination, hunger, accident or comorbidity and some even committed suicide. A telephonic survey of more than 3000 migrants from north-central India by Jan Sahas (2020) shows that majority of the workers were the daily wage earners and at the time of lockdown, 42% were left with no ration, one third was stuck at destinations city with no access to food, water and money, 94% don't have worker's identity card (Jan Sahas, 2020). Sudden lockdown also stranded many migrants in different cities of the country. Those who were travelling were stuck up at stations or state or district borders. Many were forced to walk hundreds of miles on foot to reach their home villages finding no public transport. Those who reached their native villages were seen as potential carriers of the infection and were ill-treated by the police and locals. In one of the instances, a group of returnees were sprayed with chemicals to disinfect them for which the local administration apologized (India Today, 2020). This is one of the biggest streams of mass return migration in the country. The very effort to stave off the pandemic turned into one of the greatest human tragedy in India's recent history.

Coronavirus outbreak can lead to a loss of livelihood for those who either work on short-term contracts or those who are without any job contracts. This includes several jobs in different industries. For example, in the tourism industry, guide, employees of parking contractors, cleaners, waiters in restaurants, suppliers of vegetables and flowers to the hotels and so on. A similar scenario would likely to prevail in other industries (like manufacturing and non-manufacturing) mainly because of the falling demand. Manufacturing industries such as cement, plastics, rubber, food products and textiles would reduce substantial jobs. The transportation sector is also badly affected. This will lead to the cut down of the job market (especially those who are employed) and also make hardship for job creation. Besides, this will also have an effect on pay-cuts and late increments. India is likely to face the job crisis because of the COVID 19. Migrant workers and workers in the informal sector are likely to be badly hit (ILO 2020).

The most vulnerable section would be those migrant workers who are employed in the informal sector, those who do not have either security of employment or any social protection. In urban areas, average wage earnings per day by casual labour engaged in works other than public works ranged between INR 314 to INR 335 (less than $5) among males and nearly INR

186 to INR 201 (less than $3) among females during 2017-18 (Ministry of Statistics and Programme Implementation, 2019). A large number of migrant workers and workers in the informal sector just have been surviving on subsistence wages. The Coronavirus outbreak and subsequent lockdown is going to affect them badly, leading to their further impoverishment due to loss of livelihood. It may also affect their food and nutritional intake, access to health care and education of children hugely.

Immigrants and Refugees

In the wake of the outbreak of COVID-19, immigrants and refugees who are not the citizens faced unprecedented hardship in several parts of the world. The COVID-19 could be devastating for immigrants and refugees in both developed as well as developing countries. In less developed countries, having inadequate sanitation and infrastructural facilities can cause enormous strains on public health systems which can impact hundreds of millions of people, especially immigrants, refugees, internal migrants and displaced populations. On the other hand, the official data on refugee and asylum seekers in India are small i.e., 2,07,808 as per UNHCR[2]. Luckily, India has a small immigrant population, i.e., about 6 million as per the 2011 Census.

Immigrants and the refugee population are often left out of epidemic preparedness planning and reaching out these marginalized population is a challenge. In some of the middle-east countries such as Iraq, Lebanon, Syria, where the public health system is fragile due to the continuous war and political neglect, it is difficult to control the spread of Coronavirus. This is because of the large number of refugees and displaced persons having dismal conditions such as no fixed place to live; authorities might not know how to contact them or have the capacity to coordinate a response. Sometimes, there is strong anti-refugee sentiment among national authorities. There is also scarce culturally and linguistically accessible information about COVID-19 and how to protect oneself and others, which further increases the risks to refugees and migrants as well as host populations (WHO, 2020).

In the United States of America and European countries, many of the migrant workers are subjected to adverse conditions with little to no safety equipment, no social distancing and no additional support or pay (Tharoor, 2020). Britain's National Health Service reported more than 13 per cent of the workforce is a non-British nationality. The first four doctors in Britain to die of COVID-19, the disease caused by the Coronavirus, while treating patients, were all from an immigrant background (Tharoor, 2020). However, xenophobic rhetoric about how migrants and refugees are potential carriers of the deadly virus pose a health threat (Zargar, 2020). On the United States-

---

[2] http://popstats.unhcr.org/en/persons_of_concern

Mexico border, there are growing fears over the devastating consequences of a potential outbreak of the virus in makeshift camps where thousands of migrants have been encamped for months, awaiting entry into the US. With regard to South Asian Countries, the government of Thailand temporarily banned cross-border travel between Thailand and neighbouring countries. The Myanmar and Cambodian embassies in Thailand are urging migrant workers to not return home in order to avoid spreading the virus. However, the efforts were failed due to the number of migrant workers trying to exit Thailand as they have the concern that staying back without work would lead to a shortage of food (Rogovin, 2020). While some of the countries like Libya, it has been reported that Coronavirus outbreak could be 'catastrophic' for migrants. The International Organization for Migration (IOM) – a UN Agency, has warned that an outbreak of the coronavirus in Libya could be "truly catastrophic" for the internally displaced people (IDP) and close to 700,000 refugees and migrants in the war-torn country (Ghani, 2020). With the limited financial resources, overcrowded and unsanitary conditions in detention centres, non-accessibility of information about the virus and how to protect it and limited access to healthcare services gives an additional challenge during the outbreak of COVID-19.

Various countries and organizations have responded on the impact of COVID-19 on migrants and the ways to provide support to migrants. For instance, Portugal has temporarily given all migrants and asylum seekers full citizenship rights, granting them full access to the country's healthcare as the outbreak of the novel coronavirus escalates in the country (The Week 2020). The Govt. of Malaysia has advised the illegal migrants or foreigners without travelling documents, including the Rohingyas to come forward for COVID-19 screening test (Daud, 2020). Migrants in Thailand are entitled to COVID-19 screening and treatment regardless of legal status, with documented workers covered by the Migrant Health Insurance Scheme or the Social Security Fund. Those who are registered under the Social Security Fund are also entitled to benefits for loss of income due to the government order to suspend employment in certain sectors.

Emigrants and Returnees

India is a leading country of origin of international migrants with about 17 million emigrants according to the latest estimates released by the United Nations (2019). India also continues to be the top remittance (USD 78.6 billion) recipient country as well (World Migration Report 2020). Every year a large number of people from India go abroad for overseas employment purposes. Some of the major destination countries of Indian emigrants are United States of America, Malaysia, Saudi Arabia, U.A.E, United Kingdom, South Africa, Canada, Singapore, Kuwait, Oman, Qatar, Thailand, and New

Zealand. Although a number of skilled/semi-skilled workers, students and highly skilled professionals move to countries such as USA, UK, Canada, Australia etc., where labour and employment laws are well defined and emigrants' interests are well protected under the local law, a considerable proportion of the emigrants from India are less educated and less or semi-skilled workers migrating to Gulf countries. Kerala tops the emigration rate among major Indian states followed by Punjab, Tamil Nadu, and Andhra Pradesh (including Telangana) (Bhagat *et al.*, 2013). These are the states badly hit by COVID-19. In some of the Gulf countries, many Indian migrants are locked down in a crowded neighbourhood, raising fears it will become a coronavirus hotbed while some other countries have asked the migrant workers to stay home, and stopped paying them. The lockdown imposed in many of the gulf countries has dramatically slowed their economies. This loss will affect not only the workers but also the respective state economies (The Indian Express, 2020).

COVID-19 has brought into sharp focus the international migrants from India and the major migration corridors India shares with the world. Many of the developed countries such as the United States of America, Spain, Italy, United Kingdom, Germany have witnessed an exponential increase in the number of COVID 19 cases during the past few days. Govt of India has rescued many emigrants from these affected countries prior to the lockdown in India (First Post, 2020). Many are likely to return after the lockdown is lifted either due to jobless or to prevent such agonies from happening in the future.

Response of the Central and State Governments

The spread of the Coronavirus Disease 2019 (COVID-19) and subsequent nationwide lockdown to control its further outbreak brought turmoil in the lives of millions who are primarily involved in the informal sector. To mitigate the effect of the lockdown on the vulnerable groups, Government of India on 26 March 2020, announced a INR 1.70-lakh-crore package under the *Pradhan Mantri Gareeb Kalyan Yojana*. It has within its ambit health workers, farmers, wage workers, economically vulnerable categories, especially women, elderly, and unorganised-sector workers, Jan Dhan account holders and Ujjwala beneficiaries. The scheme entails an additional 5 kg of wheat or rice and 1 kg of preferred pulses every month to 80 crore beneficiaries for the next three months. Central Government also gave an order to the state governments to use Building and Construction Workers Welfare Fund of INR 52,000 crores to provide relief to Construction Workers through direct benefit transfer (DBT) (DHNS, 2020; Government of India, 2020a). The PM Cares Fund also allocated 1,000 crore to the state governments to meet the expenses of food, travel and shelter of migrant workers. The Reserve Bank of India (RBI) also joined later with a sharp cut of interest rate along with a series of unconventional measures to lend to besieged businesses (Bloomberg Quint, 2020).

However, the fear of loss of livelihood sparked into the mass exodus of millions of these migrant labourers in some parts of the country, who started on a long 'barefoot' journey with their families, in the absence of the transportation facilities, to their native places (Bindra and Sharma, 2020). Looking at the gravity of the situation, many states, i.e. Delhi, Uttar Pradesh, Rajasthan, Bihar, and Karnataka arranged special busses to drop these workers and their families to either state borders or to their districts (Bhora, 2020; NDTV, 2020; Press Trust of India, 2020a; Press Trust of India, 2020b). This massive migration led to the chaotic situation on national highways, bus stops and railway stations and raised misunderstandings between states. As this was the violation of and a threat to the benefits of lockdown and was risky for them and for people in the villages, Government of India gave a strict order to seal all inter-state and district borders on 29 of March 2020 and asked states to issue necessary orders to District authorities to ensure adequate arrangements of temporary shelters (especially near highways) with adequate amenities and basic requirements, provision of food, clothing and health measure for the poor and needy people including migrants labourer, stranded due to lockdown measures in their respective areas (Press Trust of India, 2020c; Government of India, 2020b).

Ministry of Home Affairs (MHA) also asked the landlords not to charge rent during this crisis and employers to make the payment of wages of their workers without deduction for the period of closure (Government of India, 2020b). MHA set-up a control room to monitor the situation 24X7 to ensure the access to essential commodities to anyone (Press Trust of India, 2020d). States were allowed to utilise money in the State Disaster Relief Fund (SDRF) to provide food, accommodation and medical care to homeless, including migrant workers, stranded due to lockdown and sheltered in relief camps and other places (Joy and DHNS, 2020; Press Trust of India, 2020c). Till 31st March 2020, 6.6 lakh migrant workers were accommodated in the 21,604 relief camps with the provision of food, shelter and other basic necessities. Additionally, arrangements for food have been made for 23 lakh persons (Kulkarni, 2020). In another order, Ministry of Home Affairs issued an advisory for health actions in places of concentration of migrant workers (Government of India, 2020c), which included the three types of migrant workers and their health risk management:

Migrant workers who are still in the cities of local residence, if they are found to be forming any congregation in bus station/railway stations or any other place of the city. Authorities should record the details of such people and follow them up for 14 days, and risk screening should be done by district health authorities.

Migrant workers who are on their way and are yet to reach their destination city/village, for them the quarantine centre were to be set-up with proper amenities and basic requirement. Thermal screening will be carried out with appropriate actions for suspected or confirmed cases. They will be encouraged to be in contact with their families

Migrant workers who have reached their destination will be identified by the district administration and Integrated Disease Surveillance Program (IDSP)will follow them up at their residence.

Government of India also talked about the mental health of these migrant workers and issued guidelines. The government emphasised that immediate concerns faced by such migrant workers primarily relate to food, shelter, healthcare, fear of getting infected or spreading the infection, loss of wages, concerns about the family, anxiety, fear and mental health. As an immediate response, measures to be taken to address these concerns and need for social distancing, adherence to protocols for management of COVID-19, putting up mechanisms to enable the migrant workers to reach to the family members through telephone, video calls etc. and ensuring their physical safety (Government of India, 2020d). In a recent report, the government has proposed to send trained counsellors and community group leaders belonging to all faiths to the relief camps and shelter homes to deal with any consternation that the migrants might be going through (Press Trust of India, 2020e) on the direction of Supreme Court.

Though the lack of proper guidelines to implement the strategies posed several challenges in front of state governments in the form of lack of preparedness, however in line with orders given by the central government, majority states have devised their own strategies and taken substantial measures to protect the lives and rights of migrants during this time. The states of Delhi, Bihar, Odisha, Kerala and Maharashtra provided temporary shelters to all the migrant workers. Many states like Delhi, Uttar Pradesh, Odisha, Kerala, Telangana, Karnataka are providing free food or ration bags to migrant workers, homeless and poor people along with the distribution of food grain kits. Many municipal corporations also have taken the initiative to assist migrants and stranded people by starting community kitchen, health care to migrants, providing awareness to them and collecting funds to support the needy. For instance, in Kerala, as some of the migrants have issues in understanding the local language, police officers identified home guards who could speak Hindi, and they were given responsibility to create awareness among the migrants regarding the disease, its prevention and also migrants were ensured that the government would provide all the support to them. In Kerala, apart from food and accommodation, entertainment facilities have also been provided in some of the shelters/camps. Several states, including Uttar Pradesh and Bihar, have already announced major relief measures using DBT for expedient transmission. The governments of Delhi, Uttar Pradesh, Telangana, and Karnataka have already transferred or in the process of transferring the funds in the accounts of vulnerable groups.

States have also initiated the involvement of Non-government Organisations (NGOs), Jail mates and volunteers to support them in this endeavour. NGOs have now started crowd-funding efforts to find a way out to help those in need and they are making substantial efforts to feed people, provide them meal kits, hygiene kits, family kits of essentials. Additionally, many high-end restaurants and IT companies are also chipping in to meet the target of supply food. For instance, in Gurugram, many five star restaurants are serving food to more than 75,000 people daily (Goel, 2020) and WIPRO is donating 40,000 food packets per day. New initiatives are also taken by NGOs, for instance, in Kerala, a mobile testing unit named "Bandhu" has been introduced by Centre for Migration and Inclusive Development with the help of the government of Kerala for screening the migrants for COVID-19 and providing other medical services to the specific group. In the state, organisations have proposed to introduce a geo-tracking system with the help of the police to ensure that only migrants get access to the food.

As mentioned earlier, there are more than 200 million migrant workers in India. The inter-state migrants working in the informal sector and those who are temporary and circular migrants are hugely affected. The relief provided by the government and non-government organization may bring some relief to the migrants, but looking into the large migrant population, the amount of help is highly inadequate.

Challenges and Future Strategy

There is huge uncertainty about how long this crisis will last and what damage it would do to the economy and livelihood of people. Given its size and spread, management of migrants under lockdown and afterwards represents a massive logistic challenge. Some of these challenges need to be addressed instantly and some are in the long run:

The immediate challenges migrants face are:

- to provide food and basic amenities at camps/shelters by maintaining better hygiene and sanitation (soap/ water/ toilet/ waste management) to all of them;

- to provide the basic income support to migrants and their left-behind families who are not registered to the social schemes and depend on daily wages for survival;

- to provide basic health care and preventive kits (like mask, sanitisers, and gloves etc.);

- to quickly appraise their conditions and do the screening of the possibly infected persons and quarantine them separately;

- to maintain the social distancing for the migrants to check the spread of infection;

- to provide counselling and psychological support to the migrants under the distress

- to transfer migrants safely to their hometown: There were incidences of mass gathering of migrant labourers, violating the norm of social distancing, in Mumbai, Surat and Delhi after the end of the first phase of lockdown, reflects their desperation to go back to their families in villages. The frequent extension of lockdown has created mental agony among them. A large number have managed to return by the end of May. Hence, there is a challenge to rehabilitate them in their villages and respective native places.

- to deal with likely economic stress in the destination areas: With severe disruption in economic activities, the question arises whether reverse migrants will come back to work in towns or stay in their villages. If they don't return, how to deal with likely economic stress in the destination areas is a challenge. In the origin villages, where resources are scarce and opportunities are limited, it would be a challenge for the state government to meet the basic requirements of the people.

Governments need to address the challenges facing internal migrants by including them in health services and cash transfer and other social programs, and protecting them from discrimination (World Bank, 2020). Some of the strategies which are already adopted by the central and state government of India and various organizations, and some of the suggested strategies are as follows:

1. Several state governments are running relief/shelter camps in different states. There is no definite estimate available at the moment but not less than 10 million migrant workers are stranded. While their families at the place of origin are being supported through various measures under *Pradhan Mantri Gareeb Kalyan Yojana* announced on 26th March 2020, the stranded migrant workers are hardly getting anything except food in the camps. It is suggested that each stranded migrant worker in cities should be given INR 6000 (less than $100) (i.e., the minimum rate of Mahatma Gandhi National Rural Employment Guarantee Scheme (MGNREGS) INR 202 (less than $3) per

day X 30 days) by the Central Government in addition to the financial support by the State Government per month for at least three months. It would be advisable to give monetary support in cash to the stranded migrant workers in camps, designated shelters and other places in cities.

2. The government issued the guideline for the movement of the migrant labourers on 19th April 2020 which allows the movement of intra-state migrant labourers to carry economic activities outside the coronavirus hotspot zones, but did not allow the inter-state movement of labourers. Following the prevention and screening guidelines for the intra-state transfer of the labour is a big challenge of both the state and central governments at the place of origin and destination of migrants may coordinate with the central government and plan strategies to provide transportation to these migrants. Migrants may be screened before departure and after reaching the hometown, they should be quarantined for 14 days before sending them to their homes. Further, in order to avoid stigma by the co-villagers, awareness may be provided to villagers with the help of NGOs, Self-Help Groups, health workers and functionaries of the local bodies.

3. There is an urgent need for the development of an authentic database for the stranded migrants at the destination, in highway camps and return migrants in villages. Data on volume and characteristics of the migrants (in camps, home quarantine) is needed to transfer the benefits of social welfare schemes at present and for future management needs.

Apart from these immediate measures, some of the following long term strategies may be adopted:

1. Food grain and pulses need to be supplied on a weekly basis to meet the food and nutritional needs of migrant workers and their families. The government should use the Public Distribution System (PDS) infrastructure and distribute the food grain lying as a buffer stock to the tune of 60 million metric tonnes with Food Corporation of India. It should also mobilise local bodies to ensure the supply of daily needs arising from the Coronavirus disruption. There is a need to remember that lockdown in the West is affordable while people in India cannot bear the lockdown with an empty stomach for a long time.

2. Migrants cannot be neglected as a stakeholder in development for a long time. Integration of migrants with development is the need of the hour. The government should seriously look into the recommendations UNESCO-UNICEF and the Working Group on Migration and implement them at the earliest (Bhagat, 2012; Working Group on Migration, 2017).

3. Public health system, particularly at the primary and secondary care, needs to be strengthened, investment should be increased, drug supply and

equipment needs to be made available at massive scale, and most importantly human resources of the public health system need to be augmented a spectacular level.

4. India is a vast country with a population of about 1.3 billion. The approach of one size fits all is not likely to work. There is a need to accept decentralisation as a basic strategy of providing health services. Apart from decentralisation, the convergence of various services related to food and nutritional programmes, water and sanitation programmes, employment and livelihood programmes must be made effective. It is high time to establish synergy and coordination between the central and state government. Other agencies need to be mobilised to fight COVID 19 by taking the help of village Panchayat and Self Help Groups, and other stakeholders of society like NGOs and corporates.

5. Starting of health insurance scheme for internal migrants may be helpful for the state government as well as migrants at the destination, especially during any epidemic or pandemic. For instance, in Kerala, a health insurance scheme known as *Awaz Health Insurance Scheme*, is offered to support migrants. This scheme is also helpful to provide valid documents to migrants and helps the government to have a record of migrants.

6. There may be a large number of international migrants who might lose jobs due to COVID-19 pandemic and forced to return. Therefore, there is a requirement for the government to help those return migrants by providing them guidance, training and financial support to those who wish to set up business in order to successfully reintegrate them in the place of origin. For example, in Kerala, there is a scheme by Norka Department for Return Migrants which offers return migrants, who wish to set up a business in Kerala, a capital subsidy and interest subsidy for their investment.

7. There is a need to strengthen the database on migration and migrant households through the Census, National Sample Survey (NSS), National Family Health Survey (NFHS) and Migration Surveys. The available data are very old and also not available on time. As migration has affected the households in almost all dimensions in both rural and urban areas, an effective inclusion of migrants in our official statistics and access will be helpful in formulating robust and inclusive policy and programmes in the country.

Acknowledgement

Authors are thankful to K.S. James, P.M. Kulkarni and Tony Champion for their helpful suggestions and comments. We are also thankful to Gulshan Kumar, PhD scholar at IIPS for his help in drawing the maps.

References

Banthia, Jayant and Dyson, Tim (1999). "Smallpox in Nineteenth Century India", *Population and Development Review*, Vol 25, No. 4. pp. 649-680.

Bhagat, R. B. and Keshri, K. (2020). "Internal Migration in India", In Martin Bell, Aude Bernard, Charles-Edward, and Yu Zhu (Eds.) *Internal Migration in the Countries of Asia: A cross-national comparison*, Springer International Publishing, Chennai.

Bhagat, R.B., Keshri, K and Imtiyaz Ali (2013). Emigration and flow of remittances in India, *Migration and Development*, Vol. 2, No. 1, 2013, pp. 93-105.

Bhagat, R.B. (2012). 'Summary Report', *Compendium on Workshop Report on Internal Migration in India*, Vol. 1, UNESCO and UNICEF, Delhi.

Davis, K. (1951). *The Population of India and Pakistan,* Princeton University Press, Princeton.

Hill, Kenneth (2011). "Influenza in India 1918: excess mortality reassessed", *Genus* , Vol. 67, No. 2, pp. 9-29.

International Labour Organization (2020). ILO Monitor 2nd edition: COVID-19 and the world of work, Available at: *https://www.ilo.org/global/topics/coronavirus/impacts-and-responses.*

International Organization for Migration (2019). World Migration Report 2020, IOM, Geneva.

International Organization for Migration (2020). COVID-19 Guidance for employers and business to enhance migrant worker protection during the current health crisis. https://iris.iom.int/covid-19-crisis-response.

Jan Sahas, (2020). Voices of the Invisible Citizens: A Rapid Assessment on the Impact of COVID-19 Lockdown on Internal Migrant Workers. April, New Delhi.

Kehsri, Kunal and Bhagat, R.B. (2012). "Temporary and Seasonal Migration: Regional Pattern, Characteristics and Associated Factors", *Economic and Political Weekly*, Vo. 47, No. 4 (January 28), pp. 74-81.

Lall, V., Selod, H, and Shalizi, Z., (2006). "Migration in Developing Countries: A Survey of Theoretical Predictions and Empirical Findings", World Bank Policy Research Working Paper no.3915, Working Paper Series, May 1, 2006.

Maharatna, Arup (2014). Food Scarcity and Migration *Social Research* , Vol. 81, No. 2, pp. 277-298.

Ministry of Housing and Urban Poverty Alleviation (2017). *Report of the Working Group on Migration, Govt of India*, New Delhi.

Ministry of Statistics and Programme Implementation (2019). *Annual Report Periodic Labour Force Survey (PLFS), 2017-18*, National Statistical Office, Government of India, New Delhi.

NCEUS (2007). *Report on Conditions of Work and Promotion of Livelihoods in the Unorganised Sector,* National Commission for Enterprises in the Unorganised Sector, Govt. of India, New Delhi.

NSSO (2010). *Migration in India 2007-08*, Ministry of Statistics and Programme Implementation, Govt. of India, New Delhi.

United Nations, Department of Economic and Social Affairs, Population Division (2019). *International Migrant Stock 2019* (United Nations database, POP/DB/MIG/stock/Rev2019).

World Bank (2020). Covid *19 Crisis through a Migration Lens*, Migration and Development Brief 32, World Bank Group.

Web Based Sources:

BBC (2020). https://www.bbc.com/news/world-asia-india-52086274 access on 6th April

2020.

Bindra J and Sharma NC (2020). Coronavirus: Govt. tells SC one-third of migrant workers could be infected. LiveMint, April 1, 2020. Available at https://www.livemint.com/news/india/covid-19-govt-tells-sc-one-third-of-migrant-workers-could-be-infected-11585643185390.html, accessed on April 5 2020.

BloombergQuint (2020). Covid-19: Supreme Court Seeks Report From Government On Steps To Prevent Migration Of Workers. Mar 30 2020. Available at https://www.bloombergquint.com/law-and-policy/covid-19-fear-and-panic-bigger-problem-than-coronavirus-says-sc-seeks-report-from-govt-on-steps-taken-to-prevent-migration-of-workers, accessed on April 5 2020.

Bohra S. (2020). Jaipur mirrors Delhi scenes as '30,000-40,000' migrants crowd bus stands to get back home. The Print, March 29 2020. Available at https://theprint.in/india/jaipur-mirrors-delhi-scenes-as-30000-40000-migrants-crowd-bus-stands-to-get-back-home/390935/, accessed at April 5 2020.

DHNS (2020). A poorly thought-out package for the poor. Deccan Herald, March 27, 2020. Available at https://www.deccanherald.com/opinion/first-edit/a-poorly-thought-out-package-for-the-poor-818067.html, accessed on April 5 2020.

Daud, N (2020). COVID-19: Malaysia's illegal migrants urged to come forward for health Screening, https://www.malaysiaworldnews.com/2020/03/22/covid-19-malaysias-illegal-migrants-urged-to-come-forward-for-health-sceening/

First Post (2020). Return migration and COVID-19: Data suggests Kerala, TN, Punjab, UP, Bihar may be future red zones for contagion risk, Apr 03, 2020, Available at: https://www.firstpost.com/health/coronavirus-outbreak-return-migration-and-covid-19-in-india-data-suggests-kerala-tamil-nadu-punjab-up-bihar-may-be-future-red-zones-for-contagion-risk-8221531.html.

Ghani, F (2020). Libya: Coronavirus outbreak could be 'catastrophic' for migrants https://www.aljazeera.com/news/2020/04/covid-19-outbreak-libya-catastrophic-migrants-200403101356223.html

Goel A (2020). Posh restaurants in Gurugram turn into emergency kitchens. The Week, April 4 2020. Available at https://www.theweek.in/news/india/2020/04/04/posh-restaurants-in-gurugram-turn-into-emergency-kitchens.html, accessed on April 5 2020.

Government of India (2020a). Pradhan Mantri Garid Kalyan Package. Press Information Bureau, March 26 2020. Available at https://www.mohfw.gov.in/pdf/MoFPMGarib KalyanYojanaPackage.pdf, accessed on April 5 2020.

Government of India (2020b). Order - No 40-3/2020-DM-I(A), Ministry of Home Affairs, New Delhi, 29th March 2020. Available at https://labourcommissioner.assam.gov.in/sites/default/files/swf_utility_folder/departments/coi_labour_uneecopscloud_com_oid_14/this_comm/mha_order_restricting_movement_of_mi grants_and_strict_enforement_of_lockdown_measures_-_29.03.2020.pdf.pdf.pdf, accessed on April 5 2020.

Government of India (2020c). Advisory for quarantine of migrant workers. Available at https://www.mohfw.gov.in/pdf/Advisoryforquarantineofmigrantworkers.pdf, accessed on April 5 2020.

Government of India (2020d). Psychological Issues among Migrants during COVID-19. Available at https://www.mohfw.gov.in/pdf/RevisedPsychosocialissuesofmigrants COVID19.pdf, accessed on April 5 2020.

India Today (2020). https://www.indiatoday.in/india/story/coronavirus-migrants-sprayed-with-disinfectants-on-road-in-up-bareily-dm-assures-action-1661371-2020-03-30.

IOM (2020). IOM strategic preparedness and response plan—coronavirus disease 2019 https://www.iom.int/sites/default/files/country_appeal/file/iom_covid19_appeal_2020_final_0.pdf.

Joy S., & DHNS (2020). Coronavirus: MHA tells states to set up relief camps along highways for migrant workers. Deccan Hearld, Mar 28 2020, Available at https://www.deccanherald.com/national/national-politics/coronavirus-mha-tells-states-to-set-up-relief-camps-along-highways-for-migrant-workers-818637.html, accessed on April 5 2020.

Kulkarni S (2020). 6.6 lakh migrant workers in more than 21,000 camps: Centre Sagar. Deccan Herald, March 31 2020. Available at https://www.deccanherald.com/national/66-lakh-migrant-workers-in-more-than-21000-camps-centre-819809.html, accessed on April 5, 2020.

NDTV (2020). Bleach Sprayed On Migrants in UP Over COVID-19, Kerala Uses Soap Water (March 30, 2020). Available at https://www.ndtv.com/india-news/coronavirus-india-lockdown-disinfectant-sprayed-on-migrants-on-return-to-up-shows-shocking-video-2202916, accessed on April 5 2020.

Press Trust of India (2020a). Coronavirus: Haryana government provides over 800 buses to UP to ferry migrant workers to their villages. Deccan Herald, MAR 29 2020. Available at https://www.deccanherald.com/national/north-and-central/coronavirus-haryana-government-provides-over-800-buses-to-up-to-ferry-migrant-workers-to-their-villages-818917.html, accessed on April 5 2020.

Press Trust of India (2020b). Covid-19: UP government arranges 1,000 buses to ferry stranded migrant labourers. Business Standard, March 28, 2020. Available at https://www.business-standard.com/article/current-affairs/covid-19-up-govt-arranges-1-000-buses-to-ferry-stranded-migrant-labourers-120032800468_1.html, accessed on April 5 2020.

Press Trust of India (2020c). Coronavirus: MHA changes rules, State Disaster Relief Fund to be used to give food, shelter for migrant workers. Deccan Herald, 27th March 2020. Available at, https://www.deccanherald.com/national/coronavirus-mha-changes-rules-state-disaster-relief-fund-to-be-used-to-give-food-shelter-for-migrant-workers-818579.html, accessed on April 5 2020.

Press Trust of India (2020d). Coronavirus: Centre asks states to arrange food, shelter for migrant workers. Deccan Herald, March 26th 2020. Available at https://www.deccanherald.com/national/coronavirus-centre-asks-states-to-arrange-food-shelter-for-migrant-workers-817995.html, accessed on April 5 2020.

Press Trust of India (2020e). Take actions for redressal of migrant labourers' grievances during lockdown: Health Secretary to states. Deccan Herald, Apr 01 2020. Available at https://www.deccanherald.com/national/take-actions-for-redressal-of-migrant-laburers-grievances-during-lockdown-health-secretary-to-states-820164.html, accessed on April 5 2020.

Rogovin, K, International Labor Rights Forum (2020). COVID-19 Impact on Migrant Workers in Thailand, March 27, 2020, https://laborrights.org/blog/202003/covid-19-impact-migrant-workers-thailand.

Tharoor, I (2020). Migrants are the unsung heroes of the pandemic – https://www.wctrib.com/opinion/5030551-Ishaan-Tharoor-Migrants-are-the-unsung-heroes-of-the-pandemic

The Economic Times (2019). At 17.5 million, Indian diaspora largest in the world : UN report , 18th September 2019, Available at https://economictimes.indiatimes.com/nri/nris-in-news/at-17-5-million-indian-diaspora-largest-in-the-world-un-report/articleshow/71179163.cms?utm_source=contentofinterest&utm_medium=text&utm_campaign=cppst

The Indian Express (2020). Coronavirus deepens struggles for migrant workers in Gulf countries, 14th April 2020, Available at: https://indianexpress.com/article/coronavirus/coronavirus-deepens-struggles-for-migrants-in-persian-gulf-6361636/

The Week (2020) www.theweek.in/news/world/2020/04/01/portugal-gives-migrants-full-citizenship-rights-to-avail-covid-19-treatment.html

World Health Organization (2020). Refugee and migrant health in the COVID-19 response, The Lancet, Published online March 31, 2020, https://doi.org/10.1016/S0140-6736(20)30791-1.

CHAPTER 15

THE FUTURE OF MOBILITY IN A POST PANDEMIC WORLD: FORCED MIGRATION AND HEALTH

Monette Zard and Ling San Lau[1]

Introduction

The COVID-19 pandemic has profoundly challenged long-held assumptions about the inevitability of globalization. Despite efforts by the World Health Organization (WHO) to hew to a multilateral, coordinated and rational pandemic response, countries around the globe have responded to the emergence of the novel coronavirus (SARS-CoV-2) by reflexively closing borders and curtailing mobility. At the same time, stigma, xenophobia and discrimination have surged. As we look back at the first turbulent months of the pandemic, two competing impulses are evident: a tendency to blame, exclude and foment nationalist instincts; and a more reasoned, inclusive response that addresses the needs of marginalized populations, while acknowledging that we are all interconnected in illness and health. We are at an inflection point in the COVID-19 pandemic; whichever one of these impulses is allowed to prevail, it will dramatically shape the public policy agenda, the experiences of refugees and displaced populations worldwide, and the health and wellbeing of our society.

Public Health, Mobility and the Refugee Regime

There can be sound public health reasons for limiting mobility in the midst of a pandemic. The WHO recognizes that in the earliest phases of an outbreak, border closures may be justified to slow disease spread and shore up pandemic preparedness and response efforts (World Health Organization [WHO], 2020). However, the WHO cautions that border closures are generally ineffective at controlling disease spread (indeed, a favorite maxim among epidemiologists is "diseases know no borders" (Ferhani & Rushton, 2020)) and may be counter-productive, as demonstrated by outbreaks including Ebola, SARS and COVID-19. States may be reluctant to report

---

[1] We wish to thank Sarah Guyer for her research and editorial assistance.

outbreaks transparently, fearing reprisals and economic impacts due to border closures and disruptions to trade. Border shutdowns may also exacerbate irregular movements across borders, which are far more difficult to monitor from an epidemiological perspective; and they can disrupt the movement of essential medications, supplies and personnel that are key to the pandemic response (WHO, 2020). Responding to these challenges, the WHO has promoted the concept of "Global Health Security" since the early 2000s, premised on international cooperation, shared responsibility and the idea that the national security of each member state relies on the security of the whole. This vision is anchored in the 2005 International Health Regulations (IHR), which lay out phased, coordinated and predictable steps which governments can take to respond to pandemic outbreaks (WHO, 2016).

Even during pandemics, communicable disease control and access to asylum are not mutually exclusive. Asylum is a life-saving measure upheld by international law and recognized in many domestic jurisdictions; while human rights law allows restrictions on certain rights, including freedom of movement, in public health emergencies, any such restriction must conform to strict standards[2] and respect the principle of non-refoulement. This cornerstone of the refugee protection regime prohibits the return of people to places where they may face persecution, torture or any other serious human rights abuse. States can – and must – balance their responsibilities to protect public health, while upholding the right to seek asylum. In so doing, they should employ rational, science-based public health measures such as health screenings and quarantine as required, to keep asylum-seekers, border officials and host communities safe. The UN Refugee Agency (UNHCR) has noted that nearly two thirds of European countries have found ways to manage their borders effectively while allowing access to their territories for people seeking asylum (UN High Commissioner for Refugees [UNHCR], 2020). However, global practice has been far less laudable.

Nativism and Restrictionism: The Other Contagions

At the height of the outbreak in the spring of 2020, more than 190 countries had imposed COVID-19 related travel restrictions and 3 billion people lived in countries that had completely closed their borders to foreigners (Connor, 2020; International Organization for Migration [IOM], 2020).

Yet, migration continued – albeit at a reduced level – even as the world

---

[2] Measures must be provided by law, necessary, proportionate to the risks and reasonable under the circumstances, as well as non discriminatory (article 12(3) ICCPR, (1966).

clamped down on mobility.[3] Persecution and conflict do not pause for a pandemic. Around the world, COVID-19 related border closures have trapped asylum-seekers in increasingly desperate situations without access to protection. Aid organizations in Niger, a long-time migration transit country, have been overwhelmed by requests for assistance from stranded asylum-seekers with no route forward or back (Zandonini, 2020). From early May to June, the Malaysian government reported pushing back 22 vessels carrying Rohingya refugees, using COVID-19 as an excuse; at least 28 Rohingya refugees subsequently died of exposure and starvation at sea (BBC News, 2020).

The race to close borders has been accompanied by a rise in nativism, stigma and xenophobia, fueled in some instances by leaders seeking to deflect responsibility for their ineptitude in handling the crisis. Both migrants and native-born populations have been targets of COVID-19 related stigma, discrimination and violence, including Americans of Asian and Chinese descent in the U.S., migrants from sub-Saharan Africa in Europe, and Italians and other Europeans in sub-Saharan Africa. Refugees and asylum-seekers – from Yemen to Hungary – have inevitably been swept up in these processes and suffered immensely as a result (Gall, 2020; Yee & Negeri, 2020). The playbook linking foreigners to the spread of disease and restricting immigration on public health premises is age-old, but it has found new expression in a novel disease. In the U.S., the Trump Administration has seized on fears of COVID-19 and cynically deployed public health arguments in an attempt to end asylum as we know it. A March 20th Order issued by the U.S. Centers for Disease Control and Prevention (CDC), and now renewed indefinitely, effectively bars asylum-seekers and unaccompanied minors at the U.S. Southern border from seeking protection and expels them back to Mexico and other countries of origin on spurious public health grounds. A proposed rule, issued on July 9th on a similarly weak public health pretext, grants sweeping and expansive powers to bar people from asylum and humanitarian protection, by declaring them threats to national security and possible disease vectors. It is telling that the U.S. allowed travel for business, study, trade and other "essential" purposes to continue unhindered, while shutting the door on asylum-seekers.

Looking forward, the elements of future mobility schemes remain unclear, yet whatever evolves in the post-COVID era will have profound implications for refugees and asylum-seekers. Some of the approaches being explored may leave large swaths of the world behind. We know for example, that mobility corridors are being discussed at the bilateral and regional level

---

[3] For example, the International Organization for Migration (IOM) recorded a 28% decrease in migratory flows in West Africa in the first three months of 2020 as compared to 2019, demonstrating that while migration has decreased, people still continue to move (IOM, 2020).

to allow continuous transit between countries that have already established trading, travel and cultural ties (IOM, 2020). Quite where refugees and asylum-seekers will fit in these schemes is unclear, and it is likely that economic and political ties will trounce humanitarian ones.

It is also likely that any resumption of mobility will entail new health screenings and hurdles, which will privilege certain groups of travelers over others. Testing and quarantine regimes are expected to proliferate, and the cost will likely be prohibitive for many asylum-seekers or refugees who will bear the financial burden. Moreover, the idea of immunity passports is gaining traction and being considered by countries including Chile, despite the WHO urging governments not to issue the documents due to a lack of evidence and concerns that they may increase disease transmission (WHO, 2020). Experts have objected to immunity passports on scientific, legal, ethical and medical grounds, warning that they are unsupported by current scientific evidence and knowledge of COVID-19 immunity and are likely inconsistent with legal standards and human rights protections under the IHR (Kofler & Baylis, 2020; Latonero et al., 2020). These various initiatives do not augur well for the ability of forced migrants to access protection in other countries – an endeavour that was already challenging prior to the pandemic, but which is infinitely more complex now.

Unity and Solidarity: A More Optimistic Vision

Alongside these exclusionary trends, there are also positive signs for forced migrants. In many countries, the pandemic response has been associated with increased inclusion and recognition of migrants in national health systems and greater appreciation of the roles and rights of migrants and refugees.

Around the world, migrant and refugee doctors, nurses and other skilled personnel have been hailed for their roles at the forefront of the emergency response. When British Prime Minister Boris Johnson publicly thanked the immigrant nurses who assisted his recovery from COVID-19, it was an emblematic moment. When Americans and Britons clapped and cheered daily for essential workers, they were in effect celebrating migrant communities: in New York and other hard-hit U.S. states, including New Jersey and California, migrants comprise a significant proportion of essential workers and one third of the health workforce (Kerwin et al., 2020). Beyond health care, there is increasing recognition of the fact that refugee and migrant labour is integral to upholding economies and sustaining social services, food supply chains and other vital services in both origin and destination locations.

Several states have sought to leverage the skills and expertise of migrant and refugee healthcare workers in combating the pandemic. The governments of countries including Colombia, France and Germany directly appealed to migrant and refugee health workers to assist the national COVID-19 response (Alkousaa & Carrel, 2020; McDonald-Gibson, 2020; UNHCR, 2020). In Mexico, the Ministry of Education and the UNHCR worked together to expedite licensing of qualified refugee and asylum-seeker healthcare workers (UNHCR, 2020). Countries including Argentina, Chile, France and Ireland have eased accreditation requirements or allowed migrant health providers to work in supervised or supportive capacities (Pollak, 2020; Schafer, 2020; UNHCR, 2020). The European Qualifications Passport for Refugees (EQPR), which validates and documents overseas accreditations, served as the model for a global UNESCO qualifications passport for refugees and vulnerable migrants currently being developed (Council of Europe, 2019; UNHCR, 2020).

Yet, this increased visibility comes at a cost. In the UK, the alarming over-representation of immigrant doctors in COVID-19-related healthcare worker deaths has prompted calls for an investigation (Malik, 2020). A British Medical Association poll in April 2020 found that doctors from Black, Asian and minority ethnic backgrounds (most of whom were immigrants) were disproportionately impacted by shortages of personal protective equipment (PPE) and pressured to work in unsafe environments without adequate protection (Cooper, 2020). A Lancet study showed that frontline healthcare workers from Black, Asian and minority ethnic backgrounds in the U.S. and UK had at least a fivefold increased risk of COVID-19 infection compared to the non-minority general population (Nguyen et al., 2020).

Public health professionals have warned that efforts to combat COVID-19 will only be successful if marginalized populations, including migrants and refugees, are included in the pandemic response (Lau et al., 2020; Orcutt et al., 2020). Some states are leading by example. Early in the COVID-19 emergency, the Government of Portugal granted temporary citizenship rights to migrants and asylum-seekers, providing full access to the country's healthcare services, social support, housing and financial systems during the pandemic (European Commission, 2020).

The government of Ireland has similarly granted undocumented migrants full access to health care and social welfare, while upholding the firewall principle separating service provision and immigration enforcement (PICUM, 2020). In Uruguay, the government has announced that persons of concern recognized by the UNHCR will receive national health care (UNHCR, 2020). Aruba, Curacao, Guyana and Trinidad and Tobago have pledged to include non-citizens in the national medical response (UNHCR, 2020).

Other countries have provided more limited access to healthcare for migrant populations, focusing on COVID-19 testing and/or treatment. The Government of Kenya has pledged to provide free and equal access to COVID-19 testing and treatment for any symptomatic individual, irrespective of immigration status. Spain introduced special measures to enable refugees and asylum seekers to continue to receive aid and meet their basic needs, even if they were unable to renew their legal documents due to COVID-19 (European Commission, 2020).

Excluding individuals from health care on the basis of citizenship, immigration status or ability to pay makes little sense in the face of a universal health threat, such as COVID-19. Some experts have argued that the pandemic presents opportunities to build more resilient health systems and accelerate progress towards Universal Health Care (UHC). A study by the Overseas Development Institute found that among 49 countries that achieved or made important progress towards UHC, 71% initiated the change in the context of a crisis (Samman, 2020). Pandemics, like other calamities, are fertile grounds for innovation, potentially disrupting power structures and unlocking new political will. There are early promising signs, with many African countries waiving user fees for COVID-19 testing or treatment and countries including Ireland and Spain moving to nationalize private healthcare sectors to respond to the novel coronavirus (Samman, 2020). However, economic contraction and shifting priorities related to COVID-19 may yet present significant hurdles on the road to UHC.

Even with these positive trends, much remains uncertain. Legal access to health care and other rights may not be realized if discrimination is allowed to persist or if a climate of fear deters migrants from seeking services. It is also unclear whether temporary measures enacted during the pandemic will lead to longer-term pathways and opportunities for the migrants who risked their health and lives to serve a pandemic-stricken country. For example, the U.S. has exempted farm workers (most of whom are undocumented immigrants) from lockdown orders and declared them essential workers "critical to the food supply chain," yet refused to provide guarantees against deportation. We will have made no progress if refugees and migrants are granted privileges, rights and recognition in the heat of a crisis, only to be deprived of them after, or if they are induced to take unacceptable risks that are not expected of citizens.

Conclusion

Currently, we are at a crossroads. The forces of fear, restrictionism and nativism may lure us towards an ever more divided and inequitable society. Yet our shared experience of this pandemic is a powerful reminder that, in illness and health, we are all interconnected. In 2018, Dr. Tedros Adhanom

Ghebreyesus, Director-General of the World Health Organization, reflecting on Ebola, declared that "global health security is only as strong as its weakest link. No-one is safe until everyone is safe" (Adhanom Ghebreyesus, 2018).

For more than 70 million people forcibly displaced around the world, mobility is not a luxury but a lifeline – one that is in danger of disappearing during the current pandemic. SARS-CoV-2, a virus that knows no borders, has effectively closed the door for many refugees and asylum-seekers. After the horrors of World War II, the 1951 Refugee Convention was the global community's clarion call to never again return people to the hands of torturers and killers. As nations grapple with how to reopen borders safely and plan for mobility in the context of COVID-19, it is imperative that they account for the rights and needs of people seeking protection. Overcoming this pandemic – and rebuilding our nations and our lives – requires a collective vision, a coordinated global response and a commitment to leave no one behind.

References

Adhanom Ghebreyesus, T. (2018, February 1). *Making the World Safe from the Threats of Emerging Infectious Diseases*. Prince Mahidol Award Conference, Bangkok, Thailand. https://www.who.int/dg/speeches/2018/making-world-safe/en/

Alkousaa, R., & Carrel, P. (2020, March 25). Refugees to the rescue? Germany taps migrant medics to battle virus. *Reuters*. https://www.reuters.com/article/us-health-coronavirus-germany-refugees/refugees-to-the-rescue-germany-taps-migrant-medics-to-battle-virus-idUSKBN21C2IG

BBC News. (2020, June 9). Malaysia detains 270 Rohingya refugees who had drifted at sea for weeks. *BBC News*. https://www.bbc.com/news/world-asia-52975138

Connor, P. (2020). *More than nine-in-ten people worldwide live in countries with travel restrictions amid COVID-19*. Pew Research Center. https://www.pewresearch.org/fact-tank/2020/04/01/more-than-nine-in-ten-people-worldwide-live-in-countries-with-travel-restrictions-amid-covid-19/

Cooper, K. (2020). *BAME doctors hit worse by lack of PPE*. British Medical Association. https://www.bma.org.uk/news-and-opinion/bame-doctors-hit-worse-by-lack-of-ppe

Council of Europe. (2019). *The European Qualifications Passport for Refugees (EQPR) presented at UNESCO General Conference high level event*. Council of Europe. https://www.coe.int/en/web/education/-/the-european-qualifications-passport-for-refugees-eqpr-presented-at-unesco-general-conference-high-level-event

European Commission. (2020). *Portuguese government gives temporary residence to immigrants with pending applications*. European Commission, European Web Site on Integration. https://ec.europa.eu/migrant-integration/news/portuguese-government-gives-temporary-residence-to-immigrants-with-pending-applications

European Commission. (2020). *Spain introduces special COVID-19 integration measures*. European Commission, European Web Site on Integration. https://ec.europa.eu/migrant-integration/news/spain-introduces-special-covid-19-integration-measures

Ferhani, A., & Rushton, S. (2020). The International Health Regulations, COVID-19, and bordering practices: Who gets in, what gets out, and who gets rescued? *Contemporary*

Security Policy, 41(3), 458–477. https://doi.org/10.1080/13523260.2020.1771955

Gall, L. (2020). *Hungary Weaponizes Coronavirus to Stoke Xenophobia.* Human Rights Watch. https://www.hrw.org/news/2020/03/19/hungary-weaponizes-coronavirus-stoke-xenophobia

International Organization for Migration [IOM]. (2020). *DTM (COVID-19) Global Mobility Restriction Overview.* International Organization for Migration (IOM). https://migration.iom.int/reports/dtm-covid19-travel-restrictions-output-%E2%80%94-6-april-2020?close=true&covid-page=1

International Organization for Migration [IOM]. (2020). *Situation Report—COVID-19 Response (30 April 2020).* IOM Regional Office for West and Central Africa. https://migration.iom.int/reports/iom-ro-dakar-covid-19-response-situation-report-6-30-april-2020

International Organization for Migration [IOM]. (2020). *Cross-border human mobility amid and after COVID-19* (COVID-19 Response Policy Paper). International Organization for Migration. https://www.iom.int/sites/default/files/defaul/pp_cross-border_human_mobility_amid_and_after_covid-19_policy.pdf

Kerwin, D., Nicholson, M., Alulema, D., & Warren, R. (2020). *US Foreign-Born Essential Workers by Status and State, and the Global Pandemic.* Center for Migration Studies. https://cmsny.org/publications/us-essential-workers/

Kofler, N., & Baylis, F. (2020). Ten reasons why immunity passports are a bad idea. *Nature, 581*(7809), 379–381.

Latonero, M., Renieris, E., & Risse, M. (2020). *Examining the Ethics of Immunity Certificates* (Carr Center Covid-19 Discussion Series). Harvard Kennedy School Carr Center for Human Rights Policy. https://carrcenter.hks.harvard.edu/files/cchr/files/005-covid_discussion_paper.pdf

Lau, L. S., Samari, G., Moresky, R. T., Casey, S. E., Kachur, S. P., Roberts, L. F., & Zard, M. (2020). COVID-19 in humanitarian settings and lessons learned from past epidemics. *Nature Medicine, 26*(5), 647–648. https://doi.org/10.1038/s41591-020-0851-2

Malik, N. (2020, April 6). After this crisis, remember the NHS is not drained by migrants, but sustained by them. *The Guardian.* https://www.theguardian.com/commentisfree/2020/apr/06/coronavirus-crisis-nhs-not-drained-migrants-sustained-died-frontline

McDonald-Gibson, C. (2020, April 28). Healthcare Workers from Refugee Backgrounds Want to Help Fight COVID 19. One Man's Journey Shows How that Might be Possible. *TIME.* https://time.com/5826166/refugees-coronavirus-healthcare/

Nguyen, L. H., Drew, D. A., Graham, M. S., Joshi, A. D., Guo, C.-G., Ma, W., Mehta, R. S., Warner, E. T., Sikavi, D. R., Lo, C.-H., Kwon, S., Song, M., Mucci, L. A., Stampfer, M. J., Willett, W. C., Eliassen, A. H., Hart, J. E., Chavarro, J. E., Rich-Edwards, J. W., ... Zhang, F. (2020). Risk of COVID-19 among front-line health-care workers and the general community: A prospective cohort study. *The Lancet Public Health,* S246826672030164X. https://doi.org/10.1016/S2468-2667(20)30164-X

Orcutt, M., Patel, P., Burns, R., Hiam, L., Aldridge, R., Devakumar, D., Kumar, B., Spiegel, P., & Abubakar, I. (2020). Global call to action for inclusion of migrants and refugees in the COVID-19 response. *The Lancet, 395*(10235), 1482–1483. https://doi.org/10.1016/S0140-6736(20)30971-5

PICUM. (2020). *Statement on the Upcoming EU Pact on Asylum and Migration.* PICUM. https://picum.org/statement-on-the-upcoming-eu-pact-on-asylum-and-migration/

Pollak, S. (2020, March 20). Coronavirus: Refugee and asylum seeker medics could provide "essential support." *The Irish Times.* https://www.irishtimes.com/news/health/coronavirus-refugee-and-asylum-seeker-medics-could-provide-essential-support-1.4208280

Samman, E. (2020). *Towards universal health systems in the Covid-19 era.* Overseas Development Institute. https://www.odi.org/sites/odi.org.uk/files/resource-documents/200919_uhc_covid19_final.pdf

Schafer, S. (2020). *As coronavirus spreads, refugee doctors want to join the fight.* UN High Commissioner for Refugees (UNHCR). https://www.unhcr.org/en-us/news/stories/2020/5/5ebd461d4/coronavirus-spreads-refugee-doctors-want-join-fight.html?query=health%20workers

UN High Commissioner for Refugees [UNHCR]. (2020). *Refugee health workers step up for coronavirus response in Latin America.* UN High Commissioner for Refugees (UNHCR). https://www.unhcr.org/en-us/news/briefing/2020/4/5ea294b44/refugee-health-workers-step-coronavirus-response-latin-america.html?query=health%20workers

UN High Commissioner for Refugees [UNHCR]. (2020). *The Impact of COVID-19 on Stateless Populations: Policy Recommendations and Good Practices.* UN High Commissioner for Refugees (UNHCR). https://www.refworld.org/docid/5eb2a72f4.html

UN High Commissioner for Refugees [UNHCR]. (2020). *COVID-19 and mixed population movements: Emerging dynamics, risks and opportunities.* UN High Commissioner for Refugees (UNHCR) and the International Organization for Migration (IOM). https://www.refworld.org/docid/5ec4e2c84.html

World Health Organization [WHO]. (2016). *International Health Regulations (2005) (Third Edition).* World Health Organization. https://www.who.int/ihr/publications/978924 1580496/en/

World Health Organization [WHO]. (2020). *Updated WHO recommendations for international traffic in relation to COVID-19 outbreak.* World Health Organization. https://www.who.int/news-room/articles-detail/updated-who-recommendations-for-international-traffic-in-relation-to-covid-19-outbreak

World Health Organization [WHO]. (2020). *"Immunity passports" in the context of COVID-19* [Scientific Brief]. World Health Organization. https://www.who.int/news-room/commentaries/detail/immunity-passports-in-the-context-of-covid-19

Yee, V., & Negeri, T. (2020, June 28). African Migrants in Yemen Scapegoated for Coronavirus Outbreak. *The New York Times.* https://www.nytimes.com/2020/06/28/world/middleeast/coronavirus-yemen-african-migrants.html?referringSource=articleShare

Zandonini, G. (2020, April 9). Hundreds of migrants stuck in Niger amid coronavirus pandemic. *Al Jazeera.* https://www.aljazeera.com/news/2020/04/hundreds-migrants-stuck-niger-coronavirus-pandemic-200409131745319.html.

CHAPTER 16

MULTILATERALISM FOR MOBILITY: INTERAGENCY COOPERATION IN A POST-PANDEMIC WORLD[1]

Daniel Naujoks

The last decade has seen considerable growth in multilateral approaches to human mobility. A host of partnerships among international organizations have come into existence on human mobility, a term that refers to the broad spectrum of movements associated with migration and displacement. Since the landmark first High-level Dialogue on International Migration and Development, held at the United Nations General Assembly in 2006, collaborations between multilateral organizations have increased continuously, both in terms of quantity and quality. The COVID-19 pandemic, with its global and wide-reaching impacts on virtually all aspects of life, has affected these modes of cooperation and will continue to do so in the future. To understand future scenarios of interagency cooperation on human mobility, this chapter outlines the structural determinants influencing such partnerships. This includes structures put in place before the beginning of the pandemic, lessons from the immediate response to COVID-19, and a projection of how future features may impact cooperation in the times ahead (Figure 16.1). Due to constraints in space and scope, this essay limits the exploration to a systemic level of analysis[2] and to collaborations between international organizations, especially among UN entities.[3] The role of international organizations is important. While the real impact of international organizations is being scrutinized, Weiss (2011, Chapter 2) uses the counterfactual of a world without the UN and its ideas to show that multilateral organizations have influenced key norms and outcomes that have

[1] I benefitted from insightful comments and suggestions by Jonathan Prentice, Elaine McGregor, Riad Meddeb, Irena Vojáčková-Sollorano, Valentina Mele, Luca Renda, Nigina Khaitova, and Kristin Adina Klein. For excellent research assistance, I thank Luz Gil.
[2] For more on systemic analysis of international regimes, see Keohane (1982).
[3] This includes UN agencies, funds, and programs, as well as related organizations.

changed the world.

This essay briefly unpacks five key dimensions of interagency cooperation. It then highlights structural factors and trends for interagency collaboration on human mobility and discusses the impact of the pandemic for future partnerships.

Figure 16.1. Systemic factors determining cooperation between international organizations on human mobility

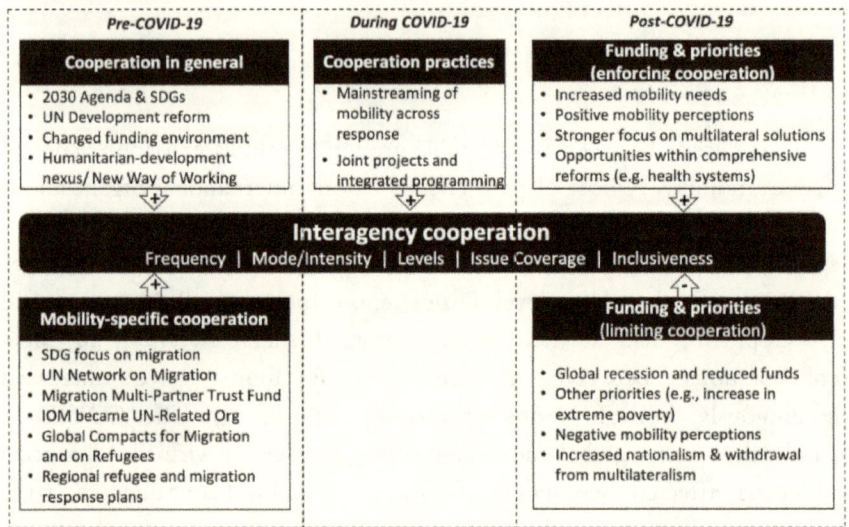

Pre-COVID-19	During COVID-19	Post-COVID-19
Cooperation in general	**Cooperation practices**	**Funding & priorities (enforcing cooperation)**
• 2030 Agenda & SDGs • UN Development reform • Changed funding environment • Humanitarian-development nexus/ New Way of Working	• Mainstreaming of mobility across response • Joint projects and integrated programming	• Increased mobility needs • Positive mobility perceptions • Stronger focus on multilateral solutions • Opportunities within comprehensive reforms (e.g. health systems)

Interagency cooperation
Frequency | Mode/Intensity | Levels | Issue Coverage | Inclusiveness

Mobility-specific cooperation		**Funding & priorities (limiting cooperation)**
• SDG focus on migration • UN Network on Migration • Migration Multi-Partner Trust Fund • IOM became UN-Related Org • Global Compacts for Migration and on Refugees • Regional refugee and migration response plans		• Global recession and reduced funds • Other priorities (e.g., increase in extreme poverty) • Negative mobility perceptions • Increased nationalism & withdrawal from multilateralism

Source: Author.
Note: +/- in the arrows indicate a positive or negative effect on interagency cooperation, respectively.

The pre-pandemic foundations for cooperation

The system of international organizations is characterized by a high degree of fragmentation (Karns, Mingst and Stiles, 2015). It includes a multitude of UN entities, Bretton Woods institutions – the World Bank and the International Monetary Fund (IMF) –, the Organisation for Economic Co-operation and Development (OECD), regional organizations, such as the African Union, Economic Community of West African States (ECOWAS) or the Association of Southeast Asian Nations (ASEAN) and many more. Several institutions and mechanisms at the global, regional and country level aim at addressing the threat of incoherent approaches, avoiding that different actors work at cross purposes, or increasing synergies between entities and activities.

Interagency cooperation can be measured in five main dimensions. The

(1) frequency of cooperation, (2) the mode or intensity of cooperation, (3) the level of cooperation, especially whether cooperation takes place at the headquarters, regional, national or sub-national level, (4) the extent of issues covered by collaborative systems and (5) to what extent a broad variety of agencies partake (inclusiveness). The continuum of cooperation modes starts with basic *coordination*. Coordination aims at avoiding conflict and overlap between the activities of different actors. It is often limited to sharing information in institutional working groups. *Cooperation* or *collaboration* involves a higher intensity partnership that enhances the activities through the buy-in, resources, and expertise of the involved actors. The mode with the highest interaction intensity is based on full-fledged *joint, integrated programming* that creates synergies between the unique strengths of the involved partners.

Truly integrated programmes between international organizations are still an exception and we lack a thorough understanding of the factors that impede or enable more and better collaboration.[4] Changes in cooperation could take place in any of the dimensions outlined above. And while we might see increases in some dimensions, other might decrease. However, this short analysis is limited to highlighting how the response to the global COVID-19 crisis and expected changes in funding and mobility priorities in its aftermath will influence interagency cooperation. As this essay cannot examine the specific effects on the frequency, modes, levels, issue-coverage, and inclusiveness of interagency cooperation, I will use *cooperation* or *collaboration* as general terms that may include a variety of the above modes and dimensions.

General trends and factors influencing inter-agency cooperation

The response to the COVID-19 pandemic comes on the heels of a number of reform processes that will continue to shape interagency cooperation. These include the 2030 Agenda and its Sustainable Development Goals that require integrated approaches across a broad range of sectors and stakeholders (Monkelbaan 2019). Since the beginning of conceptualizing the United Nations Development Assistance Frameworks (UNDAFs) and the 'Delivering as One' approach, several UN reforms aimed to bring more meaningful cooperation to the fragmented UN country teams (Mele and Cappellaro 2018). The internal guidance on the United Nations Sustainable Development Cooperation Framework – as the revamped UNDAFs are labelled now – stresses that the "2030 Agenda for Sustainable

---

[4] While cooperation between states has received considerable attention (Barnett and Finnemore 1999; Barrett 2007: Wivel and Paul 2019), the literature on interagency cooperation, especially at the country level, is still nascent. Based on an analysis of the UN framework to 'deliver as one,' Mele and Cappellaro (2018) identify two coordinating practices that help overcome limitations of inter-UN-agency cooperation, namely, *systemic thinking* and *jointly mobilizing resources* and consensus.

Development demands a UN development system that is agile, cohesive and responsive to a country's priorities and people's needs" (United Nations 2019, 4). To this end, the Sustainable Development Cooperation Framework is placed at the heart of the latest reform, as the UN Development System's collective offer to support countries in addressing key SDG priorities and gaps (p.5). The framework is meant to trigger a review of the UN country team configuration to ensure it has the capacities to deliver and comes with new tools for coordination and accountability (ibid.). Thus, it envisions that UN entities "contribute their expertise, tools and platforms in a coherent, integrated and synergistic manner" (para 9). Lastly, while the collaboration across the UN working between country offices was institutionally limited, the reform specifically aims at identifying opportunities for cross-border dialogue and collaboration, which is particularly important for human mobility issues. While there are many reasons why actual collaborations may fall short of these lofty aspirations, the reform illustrates the system's tendency toward more cooperation between its entities.[5]

In 2016, the UN system renewed its ambition to bridge the so-called 'humanitarian-development divide' (Grandi 2016). In fact, the 2016 World Humanitarian Summit established a 'New Way of Working' that is supposed to move beyond traditional silos, and work across mandates, sectors and institutional boundaries to work on the basis of joint problem statements, identify and coordinate collective outcomes, and draw on the comparative advantage of specific actors. Although for the time being, these objectives remain more aspirations than practice, the New Way of Working creates incentive structures for international organizations to cooperate, especially on refugees and other forcibly displaced populations (Hanatani, Gómez and Kawaguchi 2018).[6]

Foundations for mobility-specific cooperation

Echoing the general trend toward more meaningful collaboration, several normative, institutional and operational developments incentivize closer partnerships among international organizations and UN agencies when it comes to human mobility.[7]

First, the SDGs contain a number of explicit references to migration. This includes the necessity to protect migrant workers' labour rights, facilitate

---

[5] In addition, fundings structures are key determinants for cooperation. Whereas many donors prefer earmarked fundings and venue shopping, there is tendency to shift away from earmarked fundings and increase competion foor funds. The new, more complex funding environment is another key factor in favor of more partnerships.

[6] In some cases, progress has been under the New Way of Working, see Center on International Cooperation 2019).

[7] For the role of international organizations in the global governance of migration, see Newland (2010); Betts (2011) and Geiger and Pécoud (2014).

orderly, safe, regular and responsible migration, reduce the transaction costs of migrant remittances, as well as establish scholarships that can affect student mobility and eliminate trafficking in persons.[8]

Second, the adoption of the UN Global Compact for Safe, Orderly and Regular Migration (GCM) and the Global Compact on Refugees (GCR) in 2018 provide strong incentives for closer interagency cooperation. Within its objective 23 to "strengthen international cooperation and global partnerships," the GCM stresses that "we require concerted efforts at global, regional, national and local levels, including a coherent United Nations system" (para 40). In the lead up to the process that culminated in the adoption of the two Global Compacts, the International Organization for Migration (IOM) officially became an UN-related organization. While the IOM was already part of several UN country teams before, this change further increases the possibilities for cooperating with other UN entities and enables the IOM to officially contribute to UN county teams' approach to migration.[9]

Third, three iterations of a migration-centered cooperation platform have intended to foster stronger inter-UN collaboration. In the preparation of the UN's first High-level Dialogue on International Migration and Development in 2006, the informal Geneva Migration Group that was founded three years earlier, transitioned into the Global Migration Group (GMG). The GMG grew considerably over the next 12 years and saw several joint publications, guidance notes and incentives to work at the country level. With the adoption of the UN Global Compact for Migration (GCM) in 2018, the GMG became the UN Network on Migration, with the objective to "ensure effective and coherent system-wide support to implementation, [...] follow-up and review of the Global Compact" (GCM, para 44-45).[10] Importantly, the Network on Migration has an express mandate from the member states, a clear focus, namely to support the implementation of the GCM, including at the country level and a stronger executive structure with important implications for the promotion of cooperation. Following the GCM's call for a Start-Up Fund

---

[8] For an in-depth discussion of the SDGs' direct migration targets and indicators, see Naujoks (2018) and Foresti and Hagen-Zanker (2017) and Global Migration Group (2017) from the applied UN perspective. Naujoks' (2019) *mobility mandala* shows that human mobility is a key aspect of economic growth and employment, health, education, democratic governance, climate change and other sectors, linking it not only to the explicit migration references but to all 17 SDGs and nearly all of their 169 targets—often in multiple ways.

[9] In addition, another underlying cause for this development was that that the earlier reform of the UN development cooperation system in 2014/2015 tended to exclude the IOM from UNCTs (McGregor, forthcoming), which would have impeded cooperation on mobility issues.

[10] The call for strong interagency partnerships on human mobility is also reflected in agency-specific guidance notes (UNDP 2016, para 58-65). In addition, since 2007, the annual *Global Forum on Migration and Development* (GFMD) and since 2013, the World Bank-led *Global Knowledge Partnership on Migration and Development* (KNOMAD) have induced a range of meaningful partnerships between different international organizations, as well as research and civil society partners.

for Safe, Orderly and Regular Migration, the UN Network for Migration established a Migration Multi-Partner Trust Fund (MPTF) as a UN pooled fund. The Migration MPTF is expected to "contribute to ensuring robust, coordinated, inclusive and coherent United Nations system-wide support to Member States in their implementation, follow-up and review of the GCM" (MPTF, 2019, p. 5).

Fourth, several regional refugee and migration response plans have led to effective partnerships, most notably the Regional Refugee and Resilience Plan (3RP) in Response to the Syria Crisis that is co-led by UNHCR and UNDP, bringing together over 270 partners in Turkey, Lebanon, Jordan, Iraq and Egypt.[11]

Interagency Cooperation on Human Mobility in response to COVID-19

In addition to individual agencies' work on mobility and COVID-19, the system-wide response to the pandemic shows a strong mainstreaming of human mobility and an increase in joint and integrated projects.

The UN's general statement on addressing the effects of the COVID-19 pandemic "Shared Responsibility, Global Solidarity: Responding to the socio-economic impacts of COVID-19" highlights the particular losses for migrant workers and the knock-on effects on economies heavily dependent on remittances (UN 2020b, 8). When urging that "[n]ational solidarity is crucial to leave no one behind," the UN stresses the need to consider age, gender and migratory status for the "[p]rotection of human rights and efforts to ensure inclusion" (p. 16). Moreover, it emphasizes the need to prioritize social cohesion measures, especially where fragility results from protracted conflict, recurrent natural disasters or forced displacement (p. 19).[12]

The UN Secretary-General's policy brief "COVID-19 and People on the Move," spells out "four basic tenets to advancing safe and inclusive human mobility during and in the aftermath of COVID-19: 1. Exclusion is costly in the long-run, whereas inclusion pays off for everyone. 2. The response to COVID-19 and protecting the human rights of people on the move are not

---

[11] Cooperation on refugee issues has also benefited from the so-called cluster approach that was adopted in 2005 by the Inter-Agency Standing Committee to strengthen the effectiveness of humanitarian response through building partnerships. Since 2013, UNHCR has developed its Refugee Coordination Model centered around a Refugee Response Plan (RRP). An RRP is "a UNHCR-led, inter-agency planning and coordination tool for large-scale or complex refugee situations. RRPs present the inter-agency response strategy and the corresponding financial requirements of all partners to ensure the coherence and complementarity of the humanitarian response" (UNHCR, n.d.). For more information, see UNHCR (2019).

[12] In addition, the statement recognizes the specific vulnerabilities of young refugees and migrants who may be affected by "limited movement, fewer employment opportunities, increased xenophobia etc." (p.18) and the need to ensure that children displaced by COVID-19 have access to education (p.22).

mutually exclusive. 3. No-one is safe until everyone is safe. 4. People on the move are part of the solution." (UN 2020a, 4). In fact, the document emphasizes that "People on the move in vulnerable situations are particularly exposed to the health impact of COVID-19" (p. 8).[13] The UN Network on Migration (2020) also jointly condemned the forced returns of migrants and reminded governments of the commitments to uphold the human rights of all migrants.

The UN's *Global Humanitarian Response Plan COVID-19* aims to raise $6.7 billion, of which nearly $1.5 billion is intended for actions under the Regional Refugee Response Plans or Regional Refugee and Migrant Response Plans (OCHA 2020a, 6). The plan explicitly recognizes

"Those who stand out as suffering the most are older persons, [...] *forcibly displaced persons, refugees, asylum seekers and migrants*, and people who have lost their sources of income and fall outside social protection systems." (OCHA 2020a, 5, emphasis added).

Consequently, it highlights protecting, assisting and advocating for refugees, internally displaced people, migrants and host communities particularly vulnerable to the pandemic as one of the three interrelated strategic priorities (p. 5).[14] To this end, the plan foresees partnerships between specific UN entities[15] to advocate and ensure that refugees, migrants, and IDPs receive COVID-19 assistance; and to prevent, anticipate and address risks of violence, discrimination, marginalization and xenophobia towards refugees, migrants, and IDPs. In addition, specific mobility objectives are included in the other strategic priorities, such as setting up a Migration Health Evidence Portal for COVID-19 to provide access to research and evidence on the intersection between COVID-19 and migration health (p. 49). Consequently, the summary of the "United Nations Comprehensive Response to COVID-19" spells out specific challenges and action needs for refugees and migrants (UN 2020d, 22-23). The prominent inclusion of human mobility in the UN's global actions needed to address the fallout from the pandemic signals that human mobility is not a second-tier priority but that it is recognized as an integral part of the required

---

[13] The Regional Risk Communication and Community Engagement Working Group (2020) established guidance on how to include marginalized and vulnerable people, including migrants, in risk communication and community engagement.

[14] The other two priorities are (1) Containing the spread of the COVID-19 pandemic and decreasing morbidity and mortality; and (2) decreasing the deterioration of human assets and rights, social cohesion and livelihoods.

[15] Groups including 3-4 agencies each with IOM, UNHCR, UNICEF, UNDP, UNFPA and UNRWA are named as leads for different outcomes. The Annex to the Global Humanitarian Response Plan Covid-19 that spells out the details of the UN's coordinated appeal (OCHA 2020b, 7-13) specifies that each UN agency involved in the humanitarian response to the pandemic is addressing migrants, refugees or internally displaced in one way or another.

development efforts.

Post-pandemic partnerships on human mobility

The above analysis shows that strong factors are moving international organizations, and specifically those in the UN family, to increasingly meaningful partnerships. The response to the COVID-19 pandemic has further heightened the role of close cooperation. While these structural determinants will continue to push for collective actions, future developments will equally depend on changes in available funding and shifting development priorities.

While the bulk of factors described thus far tend to have cooperation-reinforcing impacts, future factors may have positive or negative effects. Although migration flows are projected to fall in the short-term, migration stocks may not (Ratha et al., 2020). In terms of ground-realities, the aftermath of the pandemic is likely to further increase vulnerabilities for migrants and displaced populations. As human mobility is a quintessential adaptation strategy (Naujoks, 2019), the economic consequences may increase mobility pressures and needs, which in turn, may lead to more funding and strategic priorities on the issues. However, a global recession may also lead to decreased budget allocations to international organizations, as well as to shifts to other priorities, such as the need to address that due to the pandemic, "tens of millions of people are being pushed back into extreme poverty and hunger" (United Nations, 2020c, 2). On the other hand, calls to mount "the most robust and cooperative health response the world has ever seen" (UN, 2020a, 1) or similar reforms, bring opportunities to engage mobility-aspects.

It is too early to predict to what extent the closure of borders, increases in nationalism, economic protectionism, withdrawal from multilateralism, such as the US exiting the WHO, and a crisis of trust in forms of global governance will prevail (Krisch, 2020) or whether narrow nationalism will emerge triumphant from the crisis (Torres 2020). While these tendencies were present during the pandemic, there are countertendencies that use the crisis to fortify multilateral action. The UN Secretary-General urges states to provide the "strongest support […] to the multilateral effort to suppress transmission and stop the pandemic, […] to cushion the knock-on effects on millions of people's lives, their livelihoods and the real economy" and "to learn from this crisis and build back better" (UN, 2020b, 1-2). He emphasizes the need for a "large-scale, coordinated and comprehensive multilateral response amounting to at least 10 percent of global GDP" (p. 1) and encourages the global community to "seize the opportunity of this crisis to strengthen our commitment to implement the 2030 Agenda and the 17 Sustainable Development Goals" (p. 2). Thus, addressing the UN Economic and Social Council, India's Prime Minister Narendra Modi (2020) emphasized, "let us pledge to reform the global multilateral system. To enhance its relevance, to improve its effectiveness, and to make it the basis of a new type of human-centric globalisation. [...] the fury of the pandemic provides the context for [the UN's] rebirth and reform. " While major crisis provide a window of opportunity to pursue policy change not every crisis leads to significant and positive changes. Analyses from policy change at the national level suggests that specific characteristics of the policy regime will affect whether and to what extent change occurs (Rinscheid, 2015). As several countries are in the process of drafting national voluntary reviews of the GCM implementation, the heightened levels of interagency collaboration during the pandemic might influence the future planning of its implementation.

Lastly, the pandemic led to two competing perceptions of mobile populations. While some viewed immigrants and refugees as suspicious 'bringers of disease,' the pandemic seems to have simultaneously boosted migrants' perception in many parts of the world. Not only did immigrant doctors, medical staff and researchers provide key health services. Immigrant workers in professions that were previously not labeled 'essential,' such as food delivery, grocery stores, or agricultural workers were often applauded for their important contributions. To some extent this even led to discussions to overcome the 'skilled/low-skilled' classification of work towards recognizing the work that is essential. Lastly, the UN's (2020a, 4) reminder that "No-one is safe until everyone is safe" reflects longstanding arguments about why excluding irregular and other migrant groups from effective access to public health is likely to backfire.

Conclusion

Combined with the strong foundations for interagency cooperation and the trends towards better partnerships on human mobility, the above snapshots of key factors indicate that the COVID-19 pandemic has broken down additional barriers and reinforced collaborative systems. The above analysis has outlined key factors as they result from the letter of official strategies and documents. Of course, the reality of cooperation is often not as rosy and we need to know to what degree funding structures, donor preferences, differences in mandates and entities shielding their areas of work by mandate arguments, the role of policy-entrepreneurs and brokers, as well as politics affect the dimensions of cooperation and, importantly, their outcomes. While the new UN Network on Migration provides a stronger foundation for cooperation, it needs to address how to overcome its explicit focus on the GCM and also tackle issues that lie at the intersection with the Global Compact on Refugees and other mobility questions. However, the strengthening of interagency mechanisms in light of the COVID-19 pandemic gives hope that multilateral approaches to human mobility will increase in quantity and quality.

References

Barnett, M. N. and M. Finnemore (1999). The Politics, Power, and Pathologies of International Organizations. *International Organization* 53(4), pp. 699-732.

Barrett, S. (2007). *Why Cooperate? The Incentive to Supply Global Public Goods*. Oxford: Oxford University Press.

Betts, A. (Ed). (2011). *Global Migration Governance*. Oxford: Oxford University Press.

Center on International Cooperation. 2019. The Triple Nexus in Practice: Toward a New Way of Working in Protracted and Repeated Crises, New York.

Foresti, M. and J. Hagen-Zanker (2017). *Migration and the 2030 Agenda for Sustainable Development*. London: Overseas Development Institute.

Geiger, M. and A. Pécoud (2014). International Organisations and the Politics of Migration. *Journal of Ethnic and Migration Studies* 40(6): 865-887.

Grandi, F. (2016). World Humanitarian Summit: Addressing Forced Displacement. *UN Chronicle* 53(1), p. 16.

Hanatani, A., O. A. Gómez, and C. Kawaguchi (2018). *Crisis Management Beyond the Humanitarian-Development Nexus*. London: Routledge.

Karns, K.A., Mingst, and K. W. Stiles (2015). *International Organizations: The Politics and Processes of Global Governance* (3rd Ed). Boulder: Lynne Rienner.

Keohane, R. O. (1982). The Demand for International Regimes. *International Organization* 36 (2), pp. 325-355.

Krisch, N. (2020). Institutions under Stress: Covid-19, Anti-Internationalism and the Futures of Global Governance. *Global Challenges*, Special Issue 1. Available at https://globalchallenges.ch/issue/special_1/institutions-under-stress-covid-19-anti-internationalism-and-the-futures-of-global-governance/.

Lebon-McGregor, E. (forthcoming). 'Bringing about the "Perfect Storm" in Migration Governance? A History of the IOM.' In Pécoud, Antoine and Hélène Thiollet (eds) *Edward Elgar Handbook: The institutions of global migration governance*, Edward Elgar, Cheltenham.

Mele, V., & Cappellaro, G. (2018). Cross-level coordination among international organizations: Dilemmas and practices. *Public Administration*, 96(4), pp. 736-752.

Migration Multi-Partner Trust Fund (MMPTF) (2019). Operations Manual. Available at http://mptf.undp.org/factsheet/fund/MIG00.

Modi, N. (2020). Keynote address at United Nations Economic and Social Council, July 17, 2020, available at https://www.narendramodi.in/pm-s-address-in-ecosoc-commemoration-of-uns-75th-anniversary-550579.

Monkelbaan, J. (2019). *Governance for the Sustainable Development Goals. Exploring an Integrative Framework of Theories, Tools, and Competencies*. Heidelberg: Springer.

Naujoks, D. (2018). "Achieving the Migration-Related Sustainable Development Goals." In: *United Nations and International Organization for Migration, 2017 Situation Report on International Migration. Migration in the Arab Region and the 2030 Agenda for Sustainable Development*, Beirut: UN Economic and Social Commission for Western Asia, pp. 73-122.

Naujoks, D. (2019). The Mobility Mandala. A global framework linking human mobility, public policy and sustainable development. Paper presented at the migration research brownbag series, Center for Migration Studies, New York, Nov 6, 2019.

Newland, K. (2010). The Governance of International Migration: Mechanisms, Processes, and Institutions. *Global Governance* 16(3), pp. 331-343.

OCHA (2020a). Global Humanitarian Response Plan Covid-19, United Nations Coordinated Appeal, April – December 2020.

OCHA (2020b). Global Humanitarian Response Plan Covid-19, United Nations Coordinated Appeal, April – December 2020, Annexes (May Update).

Ratha, D, S. De, E. J. Kim, S. Plaza, G. Seshan, and N. D. Yameogo (2020). Migration and Development Brief 32: COVID-19 Crisis through a Migration Lens. KNOMAD-World Bank, Washington, DC.

Regional Risk Communication and Community Engagement (RCCE) Working Group. 2020. COVID-19: How to include marginalized and vulnerable people in risk communication and community engagement.

Rinscheid, A. (2015). Crisis, Policy Discourse, and Major Policy Change: Exploring the Role of Subsystem Polarization in Nuclear Energy Policymaking. *European Policy Analysis*, 1(2), pp. 34-70.

Torres, Héctor R. 2020. International Institutional Architecture. Could it be saved? Perspective. New York: Friedrich-Ebert-Foundation.

UNHCR, n.d. Refugee Response Plans. Available at https://www.unhcr.org/refugee-response-plans.html (accessed on July 15, 2020).

UNHCR (2019). Refugee Coordination Guidance, Geneva.

United Nations Development Programme (2016). A development approach to migration and displacement. UNDP Guidance Note, New York.

United Nations Network on Migration (2020). Forced returns of migrants must be suspended in times of COVID-19. Statement, Geneva, 13 May 2020.

United Nations (2019). United Nations Sustainable Development Cooperation Framework. Internal Guidance. New York: UN Sustainable Development Group.

United Nations (2020a). Policy Brief: COVID-19 and People on the Move.

United Nations (2020b). Shared Responsibility, Global Solidarity: Responding to the socio-economic impacts of COVID-19, March 2020.

United Nations (2020c). The Sustainable Development Goals Report 2020. New York.

United Nations (2020d). United Nations Comprehensive Response to COVID-19. Saving Lives, Protecting Societies, Recovering Better. June 2020.

Weiss, T. (2011). *Thinking About Global Governance: Why People and Ideas Matter*. Abingdon, Oxon: Routledge.

Wivel, A. and T.V. Paul (2019). "Exploring international institutions and power politics." In idem (eds). *International institutions and power politics: bridging the divide*. Washington, DC: Georgetown University Press, pp. 3-19.

CHAPTER 17

COVID-19, REMITTANCES AND REPERCUSSIONS

Melissa Siegel

According to the United Nations (2020), migrants are currently being affected by three overlapping crises due to COVID-19; a health crisis, a socio-economic crisis and a protection crisis. I will focus here mainly on the socio-economic crisis. Financial or monetary remittances, loosely defined as the money that migrants send back to friends and family members in their countries of origin, are an extremely important lifeline for those that receive them. In 2019, remittances reached a record high of an estimated $714 billion, with an estimated $554 billion going to low and middle income countries (World Bank - KNOMAD, 2020b, p. 30). Unfortunately, it looks like remittances are being heavily impacted by COVID-19. The World Bank (2020b) currently estimates a 20 per cent global reduction in remittances for 2020 with continued shortfalls through 2021.

Why is this so concerning?

Remittances are not only important for the individuals, households and communities that receive them, they are also important for the overall economy in many countries that are heavily reliant on them. While there are officially 271.6 million international migrants globally (UNDESA, 2019), there are an estimated 800 million people who directly rely on remittances (United Nations, 2020) or about one in nine people supported by remittances worldwide (UN News, 2019). On average, migrants send about 15 per cent of what they earn home and half of the money is sent to rural areas where the poorest of the poor generally reside (UN News, 2019). The origin of migrants is often concentrated in specific communities. That means that the communities that are reliant on the spillover effects and spending of remittances in the local economy will likely be more severely effected.

At the individual or micro level, some of the most common uses of remittances are for meeting basic household needs, leading to the reduction in the incidence and severity of poverty (Adams and Page, 2005; Anyanwu and Erhijakpor, 2010; Hagen-Zanker and Leon Himmelstine, 2014; IFAD, 2017). It is estimated that, on average, 75 per cent of remittances are used for basic needs (IOM, 2020). Remittances are also used for household consumption smoothing (Combes and Ebeke, 2011), diversification of income, to reduce credit constraints, to pay for costs associated with education and healthcare (De Haas, 2007; Gupta, Pattillo and Wagh, 2009; IFAD, 2017), as well as better food security and nutrition (Thow, Fanzo and Negin, 2016). Remittances are generally better than other forms of external finance at targeting those who need them most (De Haas, 2007).

At the community or meso level remittances have been shown to help reduce inequality (depending on who migrates) (Shen, Docquier and Rapoport, 2010), increase business investment (Ratha, Mohapatra and Scheja, 2011), pooled remittances have helped create community infrastructure projects (UNDP, 2009) and more.

At the national or macro level, remittances have been shown to be an important and stable source of external finance; remittances bring in foreign exchange that can alleviate balance of payments burdens (paying for imports) and increase a countries credit worthiness, as well as helping to development the financial sector more generally and allow for more access to credit at the national level (World Bank - KNOMAD, 2019).

Historically, remittances have been a stable source of external financing. Remittances to low and middle-income countries are three times higher in value than official development assistance, higher than foreign direct investment in many countries and other sources of external finance (World Bank - KNOMAD, 2020c). Even in times of global economic hardship, like during the financial crisis, remittances stayed more stable than other sources of external finance (World Bank - KNOMAD, 2020b). There are several reasons for this: The first is the reason for which remittances are sent. Many families rely on remittances to help meet basic needs, meaning that migrants abroad will do as much as possible to make sure the money continues to reach their families back home. In times of hardship, this can mean reducing their own quality of life, by working more or sending more of their savings home. In general, when there is a greater need at home, we see more remittances being sent, for instance, in times of an economic downturn in the country of origin or after a natural disaster (Savage and Harvey, 2007; Mohapatra, Joseph and Ratha, 2012). In the current situation, this will be more difficult since the effects of COVID-19 are not localized in only a few areas but is having a global impact.

Even though remittances are projected to decrease in 2020, their relative importance to other foreign flows of money is set to increase. This is because the foreign direct investment is projected to decrease even more, by about 35 per cent (World Bank - KNOMAD, 2020b).

Figure 17.1 shows the current top 10 countries sending migrant remittances in absolute terms are: United States (68.5 million), United Arab Emirates (44 million), Saudi Arabia (34 million), Switzerland (27 million), Germany (25 million), Russian Federation (22 million), China (17 million), France (15 million), Kuwait (14 million), Luxembourg (14 million). Figure 2 shows the current top 10 remittance sending countries as a percentage of GDP. With the International Monetary Fund estimating the global economy to shrink by 3 per cent in 2020, all of these major sending countries are set to be highly affected.

Figure 17.1. Top Remittances Sending Countries in Absolute Terms 2018 (USD millions)

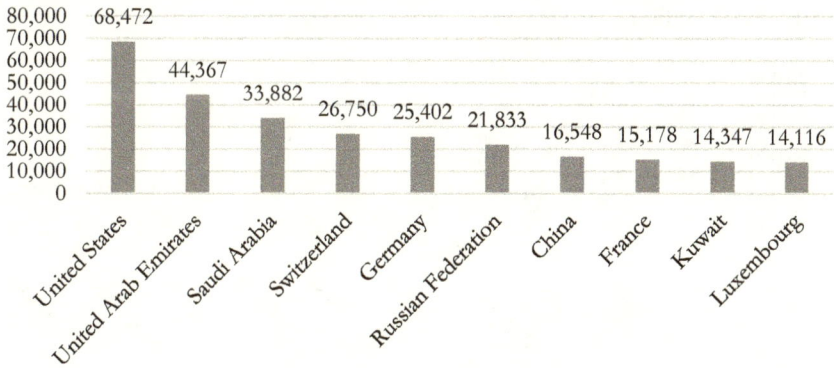

Data source: World Bank - KNOMAD, 2020b

Figure 17.2. Top Remittances Sending Countries as a Share of GDP 2018

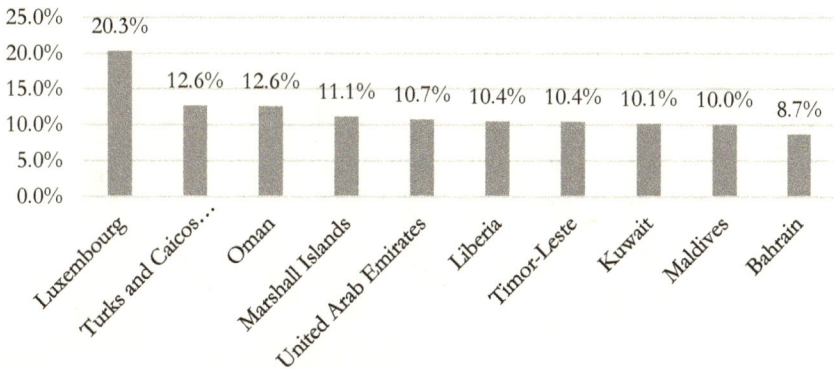

Data source: World Bank - KNOMAD, 2020b.

India, China, Mexico, the Philippines, Egypt, France, Nigeria, Pakistan, Bangladesh and Germany are the top ten countries receiving remittances in absolute terms, see Figure 17.3. Eight of these ten countries are developing countries. However, if we look at which countries receive the most remittances in relative terms, as a percentage of their GDP (Figure 17.4), all are low and middle income countries with some representing the poorest countries in the world. For all of these countries, remittances account for more than 20 per cent of their GDP. It can be easily argued that these countries are the most impacted by remittances and are, therefore, the most vulnerable during this period.

Figure 17.3. Top Remittances Receiving Countries in Absolute Terms 2019 (USD millions)

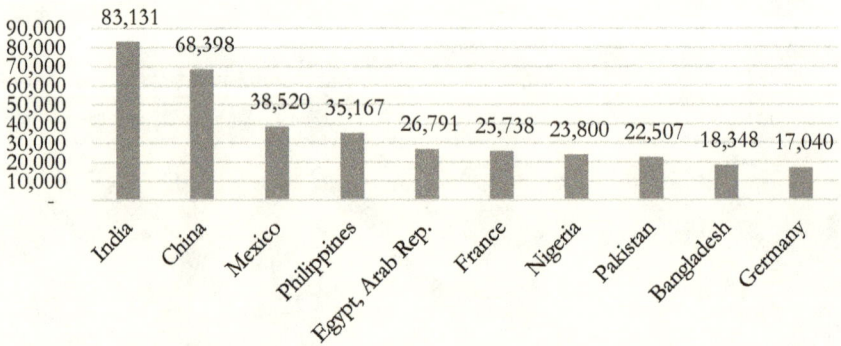

Data source: World Bank - KNOMAD, 2020b

Figure 17.4. Top Remittances Receiving Countries as a Share of GDP 2019

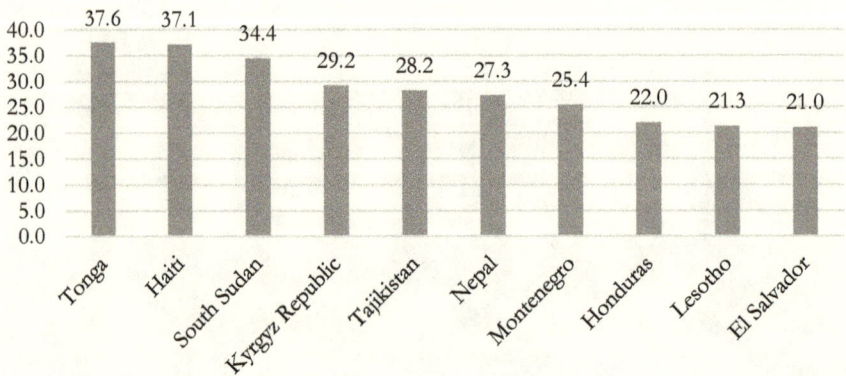

Data source: World Bank - KNOMAD, 2020b

While all regions of the world are expected to be affected by a remittance downturn, some regions are estimated to be more affected than others, see Figure 17.5. Europe and Central Asia are expected to be the hardest hit (with a forecasted reduction of 27.5 per cent). This is mainly because a large share of migrant in this region is located in oil-producing countries in the region, such as Azerbaijan, Kazakhstan and Russian. The economic down turn and loss of jobs are compounded by the fact that oil process have heavily dropped in the region meaning that these countries are likely to have budget shortfalls and a currency devaluation (World Bank - KNOMAD, 2020b). This is the compound effect of an oil price reduction and other COVID-19 related pressures are likely to be the case in other oil-rich immigrant receiving countries in the Gulf States also. Even the region forecasted to fare the least badly (East Asian and Pacific) is still forecasted to see a drop in remittances of 13 per cent. Additionally concerning, is that remittances are not forecasted to rebound quickly due to an expected prolonged recession globally.

Figure 17.5. World Bank Estimates and Projections of Remittance Flows to Low and Middle Income Regions (USD billions)

Region	2009	2016	2017	2018	2019e	2020f	2021f
Low and middle income	307	446	487	531	554	445	470
East Asia and Pacific	80	128	134	143	147	128	138
Europe and Central Asia	36	46	55	61	65	47	49
Latin America and Caribbean	55	73	81	89	96	77	82
Middle East and N. Africa	33	51	57	58	59	47	48
South Asia	75	111	118	132	140	109	115
Sub-Saharan Africa	29	39	42	48	48	37	38
World	437	597	643	694	714	572	602
Growth rate in %							
Low and middle income	-5	-1.5	9.1	9	4.4	-19.7	5.6
East Asia and Pacific	-4.8	-0.5	5.1	6.8	2.6	-13	7.5
Europe and Central Asia	-14.7	-0.3	20	10.9	6.6	-27.5	5
Latin America and Caribbean	-11.3	7.4	11	9.9	7.4	-19.3	5.9
Middle East and N.Africa	-6.2	-1.2	12.1	1.4	2.6	-19.6	1.6
South Asia	4.5	-5.9	6.2	12.1	6.1	-22.1	5.8
Sub-Saharan Africa	-0.2	-8.3	9.3	13.7	-0.5	-23.1	4
World	-5.1	-0.9	7.7	8	2.8	-19.9	5.2

Note: e= estimate, f=forecast
Data source: World Bank - KNOMAD, 2020b.

Migration and remittances are highlighted in the current Sustainable Development Goals. Paragraph 29 of the preamble clearly highlights the contribution of migration for development stating: "We recognize the positive contribution of migrants for inclusive growth and sustainable development...." (United Nations, 2015).

Goal 10c is specifically concerned with remittances, with a goal to reduce remittance costs to a global average of 3 per cent with no corridor above 5 per cent (United Nations, 2015). Currently (2020), the global average cost of sending remittances is 6.8 per cent (World Bank - KNOMAD, 2020c). The current COVID-19 situation has unfortunately slowed the remittance cost reduction process due to higher costs of operation and other difficulties to business attributed to the pandemic (World Bank - KNOMAD, 2020a).

Why is this downturn expected?

There are a number of reasons this reduction in remittances is expected. The first is the current and expected impact on migrant employment and earnings in their countries of destination. The majority of migrants are currently hosted in some of the most COVID-19 affected countries. 75 per cent of migrants and 90 per cent of remittances are hosted in and being sent from where 75 per cent of reported COVID-19 cases have been reported (World Bank - KNOMAD, 2020a). The United States, Russia and many European countries have been highly affected by the pandemic both in terms of infections and economic impacts. Employment and earnings in these countries have been highly affected by lockdowns, travel bans and social distancing measure that have heavily reduced economic activity.

Migrants themselves are also at risk of contracting the virus, perhaps more so than others because of their often more vulnerable situations and their close living conditions. Migrant workers are often housed in crowded unsanitary conditions (Chandran, 2020). Even after having the virus more under control, several of the localized outbreaks in European countries have been in meat processing plants where many foreign workers are employed and residing (DW, 2020). Migrant worker are then facing a compounding effect of wage and job loss while having to deal with infections and added healthcare costs in some countries making it difficult to send back remittances.

Even if migrants have money to send home in this period (due to keeping their jobs or using savings), there are practical barriers to sending money home. Many remittance service providers (money transfer operators), such as Western Union and MoneyGram, have been effected by lockdowns, stay at home orders, reduced business hours and social distancing measures making it more difficult for them to provide services(World Bank - KNOMAD, 2020a). Another traditional way of sending money home is through physical hand carrying by the migrant on visits home or via sending cash with others traveling back to their area of origin. Border closures and restrictions on mobility have made this more traditional way of sending remittances less of an option. The relative importance of electronic transfers/digital payments have increased during this period but many migrants and their families lack access to these types of services (World Bank - KNOMAD, 2020a).

Compounding effects

There are a number of spillover or compounding effects of remittances being reduced, particularly at a macro level. For many countries, as seen in Figures 3 and 4, remittances are not only important to the individuals and households that received them but to the broader economy, especially in countries receiving a large proportion of remittances compared to GDP. Many developing countries will see a reduction in an important source of income and tax revenue just as they are experiencing additional economic hardship locally due to COVID-19. The financial sectors in many of these countries rely on remittances as a source of deposit funding that allows for more lending (Sayeh and Chami, 2020). Because of the reduction in remittances, these financial institutions are likely to see their cost of doing business increase and their ability to lend money decrease (Barajas *et al.*, 2018). Small and medium sized business that rely on remittances will now see less remittances flowing directly to them as well as having less access to finance via formal institutions (Sayeh and Chami, 2020).

What action is needed?

There is no easy fix to this situation. Countries of destination can help by making sure migrants have access to health services and social safety nets afforded to natives as well as giving leniency on visa and residence permit issues. Some countries, including Portugal, Malaysia, the UK and Qatar have taken steps in the right direction (United Nations, 2020). More good practices can be found the "UN Policy Brief: COVID-19 and people on the move". Additionally, the global community, spearheaded by the Governments of Switzerland and the UK in partnership with the World Bank, UNCDF, IOM, UNDP, the International Association of Money Transfer Networks and the International Chapter of Commerce has launched the Global Call to Action: "Remittances in Crisis: How to keep them Flowing". This Call to Action gives recommendations for policy makers, regulators and remittances service providers. For policy makers, it is recommended to make the provision of remittances an essential financial service, to give economic support measure that benefit migrants and remittance service providers and to support the development of a scaling up of digital remittances channels. For regulators, the Call to Action recommends having banks apply risk-based due diligence measures with a view on continuing to provide banking services to remittance service providers, to consider clarification of compliance and license renewal requirement for remittances service providers during the pandemic, and to provide regulatory guidance for proportionate Know-Your-Customer requirements to be able to scale up digital services. For remittance service providers, the Call to Action recommends exploring measures to provide relief to migrants like reducing remittance transaction costs, free cash pick-up and delivery and other value added services, investing in financial education and awareness, and promoting inter-operable open systems (World Bank - KNOMAD, 2020a). These are starting points, but coordinated and effective treatment of the virus and smart economic policies globally will be important to lessen the effects of the pandemic for years to come.

References

Adams, R. H. and Page, J. (2005) 'Do international migration and remittances reduce poverty in developing countries?', *World Development*, 33(10), pp. 1645–1669. doi: 10.1016/j.worlddev.2005.05.004.

Anyanwu, J. C. and Erhijakpor, A. E. O. (2010) 'Do International Remittances Affect Poverty in Africa?', 22(1), pp. 51–91.

Barajas, A. *et al.* (2018) 'What's different about monetary policy transmission in remittance-dependent countries?', *Journal of Development Economics*. Elsevier Ltd, 134(April), pp. 272–288. doi: 10.1016/j.jdeveco.2018.05.013.

Chandran, R. (2020) '"Packed like sardines": Coronavirus exposes cramped migrant housing', *Reuters*, 21 April. Available at: https://www.reuters.com/article/us-health-coronavirus-migrantworker-trfn/packed-like-sardines-coronavirus-exposes-cramped-migrant-housing-idUSKBN22315Z.

Combes, J. L. and Ebeke, C. (2011) 'Remittances and Household Consumption Instability in Developing Countries', *World Development*. Elsevier Ltd, 39(7), pp. 1076–1089. doi: 10.1016/j.worlddev.2010.10.006.

DW (2020) 'Europe's meat industry is a coronavirus hot spot', *Deutsche Welle*, 26 June. Available at: https://www.dw.com/en/europes-meat-industry-is-a-coronavirus-hot-spot/a-53961438.

Gupta, S., Pattillo, C. A. and Wagh, S. (2009) 'Effect of Remittances on Poverty and Financial Development in Sub-Saharan Africa', *World Development*. Elsevier Ltd, 37(1), pp. 104–115. doi: 10.1016/j.worlddev.2008.05.007.

De Haas, H. (2007) 'Remittances, migration and social development', *Social Policy and Development Programme Paper Number 34*, (34), p. 46. Available at: http://www.imi.ox.ac.uk/pdfs/unrisd-remittances-mig-dev.

Hagen-Zanker, J. and Leon Himmelstine, C. (2014) *What is the state of evidence on the impacts of cash transfers on poverty, as compared to remittances*, *ODI Working Paper*. Available at: https://www.odi.org/publications/8339-what-state-evidence-impacts-cash-transfers-poverty-compared-remittances.

IFAD (2017) *Sending Money Home: Contributing to the SDGs, one family at a time*. Rome. Available at: https://www.ifad.org/documents/38714170/39135645/Sending+Money+Home+-+Contributing+to+the+SDGs%2C+one+family+at+a+time.pdf/c207b5f1-9fef-4877-9315-75463fccfaa7.

IOM (2020) *Migration-Related Socioeconomic Impacts of COVID-19 on Developing Countries*. Available at: https://www.iom.int/sites/default/files/documents/05112020_lhd_covid_issue_brief_0.pdf.

Mohapatra, S., Joseph, G. and Ratha, D. (2012). 'Remittances and natural disasters: Ex-post response and contribution to ex-ante preparedness', *Environment, Development and Sustainability*, 14(3), pp. 365–387. doi: 10.1007/s10668-011-9330-8.

Ratha, D., Mohapatra, S. and Scheja, E. (2011). 'Impact of Migration on Economic and Social Development: A Review of Evidence and Emerging Issues', *World Bank Policy Research Working Paper 5558*, 53(3), p. 205. doi: 10.21648/arthavij/2011/v53/i3/117558.

Savage, K. and Harvey, P. (2007). 'Remittances during crises: implications for humanitarian response', (May), p. 4.

Sayeh, A. and Chami, R. (2020) *Lifelines in Danger*. Available at: https://www.imf.org/external/pubs/ft/fandd/2020/06/pdf/COVID19-pandemic-impact-on-remittance-flows-sayeh.pdf%0D.

Shen, I. L., Docquier, F. and Rapoport, H. (2010). 'Remittances and inequality: A dynamic migration model', *Journal of Economic Inequality*, 8(2), pp. 197–220. doi: 10.1007/s10888-009-9110-y.

Thow, A. M., Fanzo, J. and Negin, J. (2016). 'A Systematic Review of the Effect of Remittances on Diet and Nutrition', *Food and Nutrition Bulletin*, 37(1), pp. 42–64. doi: 10.1177/0379572116631651.

UN News (2019). 'Remittances matter: 8 facts you don't know about the money migrants send back home', 17 June. Available at: https://www.un.org/development/desa/en/news/population/remittances-matter.html.

UNDESA (2019). International Migration 2019 Report.

UNDP (2009). Human development report 2009: 'Overcoming barriers: Human mobility and development'.

United Nations (2015). Transforming Our World: The 2030 Agenda for Sustainable Development A/RES/70/1. doi: 10.1201/b20466-7.

United Nations (2020) *Policy Brief: COVID-19 and People on the Move*. Available at: https://www.un.org/sites/un2.un.org/files/sg_policy_brief_on_people_on_the_move.pdf.

World Bank - KNOMAD (2019). 'Leveraging Economic Migration for Development', (September). Available at: https://www.knomad.org/sites/default/files/2019-08/World Bank Board Briefing Paper-LEVERAGING ECONOMIC MIGRATION FOR DEVELOPMENT_0.pdf.

World Bank - KNOMAD (2020a). *Call to Action: Remittances in Crisis: How to Keep them Flowing*. Available at: https://www.knomad.org/covid-19-remittances-call-to-action/documents/call_to_action_switzerland-uk_covid-19_and_remittances_may_2020.pdf.

World Bank - KNOMAD (2020b). 'Covid-19 Crisis Through a Migration Lens', (April), pp. 1–42. Available at: https://www.knomad.org/publication/migration-and-development-brief-32-covid-19-crisis-through-migration-lens.

World Bank - KNOMAD (2020c). *Remittances Data*. Available at: https://www.knomad.org/data/remittances%0D.